D0695865

plement

A DOCTOR'S GUIDE TO HERBS AND SUPPLEMENTS

A Doctor's Guide to Herbs and Supplements

ROBERT S. DIPAOLA, M.D.,
AND TIMOTHY GOWER

AN OWL BOOK

HENRY HOLT AND COMPANY   NEW YORK

The information contained in this book is not intended as a substitute for consulting with your physician. All matters regarding your health require medical supervision. Throughout this book the words *doctor* and *physician* refer to a licensed medical doctor who is trained to diagnose and treat the specific condition being discussed.

Henry Holt and Company, LLC
Publishers since 1866
115 West 18th Street
New York, New York 10011

Henry Holt® is a registered trademark of
Henry Holt and Company, LLC.

Copyright © 2001 by Robert S. DiPaola, M.D., and Timothy Gower
All rights reserved.
Distributed in Canada by H. B. Fenn and Company Ltd.

Library of Congress Cataloging-in-Publication Data
DiPaola, Robert S.
    A doctor's guide to herbs and supplements / Robert S. DiPaola and
Timothy Gower.—1st ed.
        p. cm.
    "An Owl book."
    Includes bibliographical references and index.
    ISBN 0-8050-6665-9 (pbk.)
    1. Dietary supplements. 2. Herbs—Therapeutic use. I. Title: Herbs and
supplements.   II. Gower, Timothy.   III. Title.
RM258.5 .D57 2001
615'.321—dc21   2001024842

Henry Holt books are available for special promotions and
premiums. For details contact: Director, Special Markets.

First Edition 2001

Designed by Kelly S. Too

Printed in the United States of America

10 9 8 7 6 5 4 3 2 1

CONTENTS

A DOCTOR'S GUIDE TO HERBS AND SUPPLEMENTS

INTRODUCTION

The patient was a robust fifty-year-old man I'll call Joe. Two years earlier he had been diagnosed with prostate cancer. At the time, surgeons were able to remove Joe's diseased prostate gland. But recent blood tests suggested that his cancer had returned.

I told Joe about several options that we could try to control his cancer. He had another idea: Joe wanted to take an herbal formula he had heard might cure prostate cancer. His desire to try this product made me realize that patients like Joe, as well as all consumers, need to understand the potential benefits and risks that herbs and other natural medicines might present. I guess you could say I started writing this book that day.

Just a decade ago, few Americans had heard of herbal medicine. If you felt sick, you went to a doctor, and he or she may have prescribed a drug or some other therapy. People who self-treated their illnesses with nonmedical remedies were considered eccentric. Friends might have questioned your sanity if you told them you were using strange-sounding concoctions like Saint-John's-wort, bee pollen, or cat's claw.

What a difference a few years can make. Today, millions of Americans take echinacea and goldenseal to fight the common cold. People plagued by fatigue pop a little ginseng to perk up. Has your memory begun to slip? Your neighbor may tell you that without a daily dose of ginkgo she would never find her car keys.

Meanwhile, the use of high-dose vitamin therapy continues to grow in popularity. And hardly a month passes without the appearance of a new miracle pill, such as glucosamine (to relieve arthritis) or SAMe (for depression), which captures the nation's imagination and sends consumers flocking to health food stores.

According to a 1999 survey, more than half of American adults take dietary supplements—the general term used by the U.S. Food and Drug Administration to describe herbs, vitamins, minerals, and other amino acid compounds sold in pill, capsule, tablet, and liquid form. The very phrase *dietary supplements* suggests that these products are intended to be consumed in addition to a normal diet. That explains why they're regulated more or less as foods.

But, as a medical oncologist and research scientist, I can tell you that dietary supplements have less in common with pizza and meat loaf than they do with the medications at your local pharmacy. Which brings me back to Joe. I saw him again a month later, after he had started taking daily doses of PC-SPES. This product is made up of eight herbs, including some familiar to many American consumers, such as ginseng, saw palmetto, and licorice root. Joe had developed some unpleasant symptoms, including breast tenderness and impotence. I would soon learn, however, that his condition had changed in another striking way.

As I would with any prostate cancer patient, I tested Joe's blood for levels of a protein given off by prostate tumors, called PSA (for prostate specific antigen). Rising PSA levels suggest that tumors are growing. At his last office visit, Joe's PSA measured over 20—definitely cause for concern. But on this day, his PSA had plummeted to less than 1.

I literally couldn't believe my eyes, and had to read the chart twice. What could have caused such a dramatic improvement in his condition? The only intervention I knew of that can produce that sort of drop in PSA is hormone therapy, which lowers levels of testosterone (in turn stopping growth of the tumor). But Joe wasn't taking hormones. Or was he?

I decided to learn all I could about PC-SPES. I found no information to suggest that the product contains hormones capable of lowering testosterone. But our lab later analyzed this herbal formula and confirmed that, indeed, PC-SPES contains a potent form of estrogen—the so-called female hormone. Now I understood why Joe's PSA had dropped, and why he had developed the unpleasant symptoms. My colleagues and I began a study, later published in the *New England Journal of Medicine*, in which we followed several patients in our clinic who were using PC-SPES. All developed the classic side effects seen in men who are given estrogen therapy (which is rarely used to control prostate cancer these days, due to the risks associated with it): breast tenderness, impotence, and in one case a blood clot.

The message is clear: This "all-natural" herbal product acts a lot like a drug. And PC-SPES is hardly unique. As more research is performed on the various dietary supplements in use today, doctors are discovering that many of these products can have a strong influence on the human body—which may include serious side effects, as well as dangerous interactions with other medications.

Yet, while the herbal medicines and other supplements Americans have embraced so readily may have druglike effects, they differ from over-the-counter and prescription medications in an important way. When your doctor prescribes a painkiller, or your pharmacist recommends a cold remedy, you can take these drugs with the confidence that they have undergone extensive study to prove that they're safe and effective. The FDA requires that all over-the-counter and prescription drugs undergo rigorous testing to guarantee as much.

But federal law does not require dietary supplements to undergo stringent testing. The safety and therapeutic value of medicinal herbs, as well as vitamin, mineral, and amino acid supplements, do not have to be demonstrated before these products are sold. Some of these compounds have undergone serious scientific study, but many have not.

That's why I wrote this book: to give consumers a scientist's perspective on the hundred best-selling herbs and other dietary supplements in the United States. From acidophilus to zinc, this book offers a straightforward look at what's known—and not known—about the most commonly used natural medicines in this country.

Other books about medicinal herbs and supplements you may have read are filled with vague language, such as "this herb is said to promote hair growth" or "extract of this plant is traditionally used to cure upset stomach." You won't find such uncertainty here, however. As a scientist and physician, I'm interested in evidence. Before I prescribe any medication to a patient, I always ask myself a series of questions. How do I know it works? *How* does it work? Could it cause side effects? Does it interfere with other medications?

HOW WE CHOSE OUR TOP 100

We didn't—you did. Each year, a Bellevue, Washington–based market research company called The Hartman Group asks a representative sampling of Americans which dietary supplements they use regularly. From that data, The Hartman Group compiles a list of the hundred most frequently used supplements in the United States. The hundred entries in this book are based on The Hartman Group's list for the year 1999, with a few exceptions. We felt that two categories, Chinese medicine and homeopathic remedies, were each too big and complex to do them justice within the framework of our book. We also decided that a few categories were so much alike that they could be merged into a single entry; hence, trace minerals and multiminerals are discussed together, as are blue-green algae and spirulina. These subtractions allowed us to include entries for four popular dietary supplements that did not appear on the original Hartman list, but that we think you should know about. They include arginine, chitosan, fiber supplements, and the herbal preparation PC-SPES.

I've applied those same principles to the products discussed in the pages that follow. For each compound, the following questions have been addressed:

What is it?

In the first section of each entry in this book, we try to put an herb or vitamin in context. We explain, in lay person's language, what's known about its basic role in human health. We describe the plants from which various herbs are extracted and list foods that contain high levels of particular nutrients. Finally, we detail the forms (pill, powder, liquid extract, and so on) in which the supplement is usually sold.

Why do some people take . . . ?

Here we briefly explain why and how Americans use the dietary supplement being discussed. It's important to note that very often these uses are based on traditional medical practices, folk wisdom, and fads—not sound science.

Does it work?

The heart of this book: This section attempts to cut through all the claims and hype about each supplement and explain what scientists actually *know* about it. We searched for all the information we could obtain about each supplement described herein using MEDLINE, the National Library of Medicine's database of article abstracts from thousands of medical journals published all over the world. We also checked several other scientific databases and combed through a tall stack of reference works. Our goal was to learn all we could about these products, but in particular we were looking for high-quality studies that offered the best scientific evidence. In these "gold standard" studies, scientists attempt to determine whether a medical therapy works by comparing it side by side with a proven therapy or a placebo (a look-alike pill that contains no active medicine; also known as a sugar pill). All drugs approved for use in the United States undergo this stringent testing. I feel herbs and other dietary supplements used as medicine should be held to an equally high standard.

An important caveat is worth noting. Even the most promising results from a study involving herbs and other supplements must be viewed with a degree of skepticism. That's because the purity and content of these products are difficult to guarantee. There's little government oversight of the natural medicine industry, so manufacturers of supplements operate on a kind of honor system. What they put into the pills and powders they sell may or may not be what's claimed on the package label. This situation creates an inherent problem for scientists who study herbs and supplements: How can they claim to have learned something about a product when they can't be 100 percent certain they know what they were studying in the first place?

What else should I know about . . . ?

In this section, we'll discuss any special concerns consumers should have about a given product. What are its side effects? Does it interfere with any common medications? We'll also talk about the symptoms that may lead someone to consider using a particular herb or supplement—and why it's usually unwise to self-treat them.

In regard to side effects and medication interactions, we list the major ones learned about in our research, but since many of these products haven't been subjected to adequate safety testing, it's not possible to predict all the potential risks associated with using them. For the same reason, it's unwise to assume that an herb or supplement with no known side effects or interactions is completely safe. It's always wise, however, to talk to a physician before taking any dietary supplement, particularly for pregnant women.

Bottom line

A quick summary of what you should know about this dietary supplement.

We hope you'll consult this book before taking any dietary supplement. But since we can't discuss all of the hundreds of products on the market, and you may not always have this guide handy, keep in mind the following rules before you buy—or use—any of these alternative medicines.

RULE 1: Think of dietary supplements as drugs—because in many cases they *are* drugs.

Despite the growing popularity of dietary supplements in this country, there are plenty of skeptics who believe that they don't do a thing, that when you swallow a tablet of goldenseal or ginseng you may as well be popping Pez. And, frankly, doctors make up a particularly skeptical crowd, which you may already know if you've mentioned medicinal herbs during an office visit.

But make no mistake, some medicinal herbs and other supplements can have profound effects on the human body. What skeptics fail to recognize is that these compounds may contain drugs. That's right—they contain substances that may alter the function of organ systems in your body. It is true that many dietary supplements have no known effect on humans. But some chemicals found in herbs, vitamins, and other supplements can attach themselves to specific receptors in the heart, brain, and other organs, signaling them to change the way they behave. And according to my dictionary, any chemical that does that is a drug.

In fact, as you may know, some well-known and widely used drugs are derived from plants. For instance, digitalis, a medication used to treat heart failure, is made from leaves of an ornamental plant called foxglove. So it's hardly surprising to learn that many medicinal herbs on the market also contain druglike compounds—and that these compounds may affect human health. Unfortunately, those effects aren't always desirable; see Rule 2.

RULE 2: Understand that "natural" doesn't necessarily mean "safe"— dietary supplements can cause unwanted side effects.

It's well known that many of our most important drugs can cause unwanted symptoms, often serious. That aspirin you take for a headache, for instance, can induce stomach bleeding. Since we already know that medicinal herbs and other dietary supplements contain drugs, it's illogical to assume that they're completely benign.

Yet, some companies that sell herbs and other dietary supplements seem to want consumers to believe otherwise. They hint, and sometimes come right out and say, that herbal remedies are safer than prescription or over-the-counter drugs because they're "natural."

That's simply not true. Any substance you consume that changes the behavior of an organ system in your body may also have a toxic effect. Granted, some products have no known side effects. But there are also a number of popular dietary supplements on the market that can cause annoying problems, such as skin rashes and nausea, while still others can be downright dangerous.

Ephedra is an excellent example. Also known as ma huang, this herb is used for a variety of purposes, but it's probably most widely known as a weight-loss aid. Companies that sell ephedra-based diet pills say the products "burn fat."

Scientists know that ephedra contains a chemical called ephedrine. An ephedrine molecule is very similar to that of a molecule found in a naturally occurring stimulant called epinephrine; if you compared the two under a microscope they would look nearly identical. You may know epinephrine by another name, adrenaline—the so-called fight-orflight hormone. The adrenal gland produces epinephrine in response to a threatening situation, when your body needs to gear up to do battle or flee. One of epinephrine's roles is to tell the heart to beat faster so it can pump blood to your extremities, where it's needed most, for fending off an attacker or for running.

Not surprisingly, if you take enough ephedra your heart races and you become nervous. That's because your heart doesn't care where a molecule of ephedrine comes from—ephedra or epinephrine—it reacts the same way when exposed to either form of these closely related chemicals. Ephedra can also cause blood pressure to rise, making it particularly dangerous for people who have high blood pressure and other heart problems. In recent years, the FDA has compiled a long list of reports about people who died or became seriously ill after taking ephedra.

Of course, not all medicinal herbs are dangerous. But if you're going to take any dietary supplement, take it seriously. After all, you can even overdose on vitamins. For example, consuming too much vitamin A can cause liver damage.

RULE 3: Talk to your physician.

According to a 1999 survey, less than half of Americans who take vitamins and minerals tell their physicians. And just 28 percent of people who use medicinal herbs consult their doctors first. Many people polled said they had taken dietary supplements to self-treat serious illnesses, including heart disease, high blood pressure, and diabetes.

These statistics are troubling for many reasons. In the first place, medical symptoms require careful interpretation. What may seem like a minor problem to a lay person may turn out to be an early sign of a life-threatening illness. For instance, a person with recurrent constipation might think it's really no big deal (and perhaps a bit embarrassing), certainly not worth making an office visit. So instead, that person may decide to take an herbal laxative or high-fiber dietary supplement to treat the discomfort. But these pills or powders may end up masking a much more serious problem; for a dramatic example, consider that chronic constipation is one of the early signs of colon cancer.

Similarly, self-dosing with dietary supplements may provide a false sense of security. A woman taking an herb that she has heard prevents breast cancer might not schedule routine mammograms and other screening procedures for the disease—which have been proven to save lives. In short, the easy availability of dietary supplements may tempt you to play doctor. But don't forget that old saying: The doctor who treats himself has a fool for a patient.

Your doctor, on the other hand, has the expertise to help you understand your condition and can explain all the options medicine has to offer. He or she may also be able to discuss the potential benefits and risks associated with an alternative therapy, particularly in regard to any preexisting conditions you may have or medications you may already be taking. For instance, a doctor who understands how herbal therapies work would be alarmed to hear that his patient with high blood pressure planned to start taking ephedra pills to lose weight. As mentioned above, the herb contains powerful cardiovascular stimulants that could be fatal if used by a person with hypertension. (And if your doctor hasn't read up on herbal therapies, you may want to bring this book with you to your next office visit.)

Furthermore, dietary supplements can interact with other medications you might be using. For example, patients who are at risk for blood clots are often treated with anticoagulant medications, which make the blood thinner (and therefore less likely to clot). Some herbs are known to alter the effectiveness of blood-thinning drugs, which could lead to either excessive bleeding or the formation of blood clots. Although we mention many examples of herb-drug interactions throughout this book, it's not possible to list them all. The fact is, the safety of many of these products hasn't been adequately studied, leaving gaps in our knowledge of how they act in the human body and interact with other medications.

HERBS AND DRUGS: A RISKY MIX?

Before a physician prescribes a drug, he or she must know what other medications a patient is taking, in order to avoid causing a dangerous interaction between the two chemicals. Herbs and other supplements can act like drugs, so it's no surprise that many may cause interactions when taken alongside certain common medications. Here's how: Some drugs have what's known in medicine as a "narrow therapeutic index." That means that the drug won't work as desired if the amount in the body is decreased even slightly. Or that it could cause serious side effects if levels are increased. The presence of certain herbs and supplements can alter the level of a given drug in the body. In other instances, taking an herb or supplement could interfere with blood tests used to measure levels of a drug.

This chart lists several common drugs and drug categories (most with a very narrow therapeutic index), and the herbs and supplements discussed in this book that may cause dangerous interactions if combined with them.

The chart may not include every potential drug interaction, since more study is needed to understand how these natural medicines behave in the body. In many cases, these potential interactions are theoretical, based on what's known about the chemical composition of an herb. Be sure to discuss your use of herbs and supplements with a physician, *especially* if you're taking any prescription medication.

If your doctor has prescribed . . .	. . . then avoid the following
Antianxiety medications, such as Xanax	Kava, valerian
Antiseizure medications, such as Phenobarbital	Evening primrose oil

If your doctor has prescribed . . .	. . . then avoid the following
Digitalis medicine, such as Lanoxin (digoxin), which is used to treat heart failure	Hawthorn, licorice, Siberian ginseng
Diuretics, such as Lasix or Spironolactone, which are used to treat high blood pressure	Licorice
Hypoglycemics, such as DiaBeta or Micronase, which are used to treat diabetes	Chromium, ephedra, garlic, ginger, ginseng, licorice
Immunosuppressive drugs, including any form of corticosteroid or cyclosporine	Alfalfa, echinacea, licorice, vitamin E, zinc
Iron	Black cohosh, chamomile, feverfew, hawthorn, Saint-John's-wort, saw palmetto, valerian

MAO inhibitors, such as Parnate or Nardil, which are sometimes used to treat depression	Ephedra, ginseng, licorice, Saint-John's-wort, yohimbe
Thyroid hormones, such as Levothyroid or Synthroid	Kelp
Warfarin or other blood thinners	Chamomile, dong quai, feverfew, garlic, ginger, ginkgo, ginseng, vitamin K

Adapted from *Archives of Internal Medicine*, 1998; 158:2205

Finally, many patients turn to dietary supplements when standard medical therapies aren't totally effective. This might be true of diabetics in search of newer therapies, or cancer patients looking for that elusive cure. However, turning to herbs and other supplements when a standard medicine fails may actually limit your access to valuable therapies. That's because new medical options are often available, in the form of drugs and other medical interventions being studied in clinical trials needed to prove that they're safe and effective before being approved by the Food and Drug Administration. You may be surprised to learn that dietary supplements are usually not as well tested as these experimental drugs.

DRUGS VERSUS DIETARY SUPPLEMENTS: A CRITICAL DIFFERENCE

Many consumers who choose to self-medicate with herbs and other dietary supplements say they're motivated by fear of side effects associated with prescription and over-the-counter drugs. Medicinal herbs and other dietary supplements, meanwhile, are perceived as safer than drugs, since they're derived from plants and other natural sources. Mother Nature wouldn't poison us, right?

Companies that sell dietary supplements, which often hint that their products are gentler than drugs, reinforce this perception. I would argue that, in at least one very important way, just the opposite is true. As I pointed out earlier, many plant extracts and other natural compounds contain druglike substances. This fact alone makes the "natural means safer" argument questionable. More important, though, consider the two very different paths these two categories of medications take before they can be sold in the United States.

A company that sets out to sell a new drug in the United States is required by law to follow these steps.

- Before testing an experimental drug in humans, preliminary studies are conducted with animals to determine whether it shows any effect and is safe.
- Next, phase I clinical trials are conducted in humans to determine whether the drug is safe. Initially, very low doses are used, but treatment levels are gradually increased. Doctors monitor the functioning of various organs (such as the liver and kidneys) to determine whether the drug is causing any harm to the patients. When side effects begin to occur, a safe dosage level can be established.
- Phase II trials determine what effect a drug has in humans at a safe dosage. By the end of a phase II trial, scientists usually have a pretty good idea whether a drug does what they hoped it would do, and what percentage of patients it's likely to benefit.
- If a drug looks promising after phase II trials, it is then put to its toughest test. Phase III trials determine if a drug is better than older treatments or no treatment at all. Half of the patients in a phase III trial are given the experimental new drug, while an equal number of similar patients receive either the old therapy or no therapy. This method of testing helps rule out variables that may have led to optimistic, but misleading, results during phase II.
- Finally, the company submits data from all three phases of clinical trials to the FDA for approval. This process usually takes many years and can cost hundreds of millions of dollars.

Now, consider the steps a company must follow before selling a new dietary supplement in the United States, under guidelines set forth by the Dietary Supplements Health and Education Act of 1994:

- If the ingredients were on sale in the United States before October 15, 1994, the supplement may be sold without submitting any information regarding safety and effectiveness to the FDA. Most medicinal herbs on sale in the United States today have been available here for many years, meaning they were essentially preapproved by this "grandfather" clause.

▸ If the supplement contains ingredients that were not marketed in the United States before October 15, 1994, the company wishing to sell the product must notify the FDA at least seventy-five days in advance and provide evidence that the new ingredient "will reasonably be expected to be safe." But the companies themselves—not the government—decide what constitutes adequate evidence of safety.

That's it. As you can see, companies that sell dietary supplements must meet a much lower standard to demonstrate that their products are safe and effective. Add the fact that dietary supplements are difficult to patent, and there's little financial incentive for these companies to take the time and spend the money to study the products they sell. As a result, we know much less about dietary supplements than we do about pharmaceutical products.

There's also a serious question as to whether consumers are getting their money's worth when they buy dietary supplements. Undoubtedly, many companies that market these products strive to produce high-quality herbs and vitamins. But there's little doubt that lax regulatory standards have led to sloppy manufacturing practices in the dietary supplements industry. Throughout this book we describe several cases in which watchdog groups conducted lab analyses on popular brands of supplements, only to find that they lacked the advertised levels of active ingredients. When it comes to purchasing dietary supplements, buyers must beware—of both their health and their wallets.

While there's a proper role in medicine for some dietary supplements, many talked-about and heavily hyped products simply haven't been properly studied. All too often, claims made about herbs and supplements aren't backed up by solid scientific evidence. I hope reading this book helps you to protect your health and safety by becoming a more critical consumer. If you take away no other message, let it be this: Any chemical you consume that can alter the way your body functions is a drug, no matter what the package label says.

In a broader sense, I hope you'll come to see why the worlds of conventional medicine and alternative therapies should no longer be viewed as somehow separate and distinct. There's only one kind of medicine that matters, after all—the kind that has been thoroughly tested and proven to be safe and effective.

PACKAGE LABELS, DECODED

The dietary supplements industry receives little government oversight, but it has to accept a trade-off for this freedom. Federal law limits what sellers of dietary supplements can claim about their products. Specifically, they're not permitted to state on package labels or in ads that their products may be used to diagnose, treat, cure, or prevent any disease. Drug sellers, on the other hand, are permitted to make such claims. However, makers of dietary supplements are allowed to claim that their products may have an effect on the "structure or function" of the human body. Many critics feel this is a rather fuzzy distinction. But think of it this way: The label on a dietary supplement cannot say "prevents heart disease," but it can bear the phrase "supports cardiovascular health." Likewise, the statement "cures arthritis" is off-limits, but "promotes strong joints" is not.

A wise consumer always reads the entire package label before using any product as medicine or to improve health. But if you've ever shopped for dietary supplements, you're probably familiar with the suggestive, if curiously vague, language often found on package labels. The chart will help you learn how to decode the claims on supplement labels—and show why you should be particularly cautious when you see certain phrases.

If it says . . .	. . . then beware
"Treats symptoms of menopause"	This product may contain estrogens, which could increase the risk of several types of cancer, particularly uterine cancer.
"Improves mood," "promotes a sense of well-being," and "relieves anxiety"	May contain Saint-John's-wort, which could interact with several common medications. Or it may contain a relaxant, such as valerian or kava—driving a car or operating heavy machinery while using this herb could prove dangerous.

"Promotes circulation"	May contain any of several herbs that purportedly increase blood flow, which could alter the effect of anticoagulant medications.
"Burns fat" or "boosts energy"	May contain ephedra or some other substance that acts as a cardiovascular stimulant—which may be dangerous.
"For regularity," "colon conditioner," or "removes toxins"	Probably contains a laxative; abuse could lead to dependence and other health problems.
"For prostate health"	May contain estrogen-like substances that could decrease testosterone levels and lead to blood clots and other serious health risks.
"Contains antioxidants"	Claims about these substances—which include beta carotene, vitamin E, selenium, vitamin C, and others—aren't necessarily backed by scientific evidence, although further study may prove that some have health benefits. However, some antioxidants (such as beta carotene) may actually be *harmful* to some people.

WHAT ARE FUNCTIONAL FOODS?

Not long ago, when people talked about "health food," they were often referring to conventional edibles that had some or all of an unhealthy component—fat, sugar, or salt, usually—removed. Think of fat-free frozen yogurt and low-sodium soups, for instance. Today, a new generation of products filling grocers' shelves has reversed that trend. So-called functional foods are familiar products containing added ingredients that allegedly improve health. These new foods run the gamut from orange juice with added calcium to tortilla chips sprayed with Saint-John's-wort. According to *Nutrition Business Journal*, by 2010 Americans may spend up to $50 billion a year on functional foods.

But should we? Only a few of these foods have been studied. One example is the margarine known as Benecol, which has an added compound known as sitostanol (which is derived from pine oil and other sources). Several studies have shown that Benecol lowers cholesterol when consumed as part of a low-fat, low-cholesterol diet. (However, it is still not clear whether this product is safe for long-term use, or if it's as effective as other proven interventions.) Some functional food and beverages contain added calcium and fiber. Studies show that increasing your intake of these nutrients may have health benefits, while conferring minimal risk of side effects (though you should still talk to a doctor before adding these products to your diet).

Of greater medical concern is the trend toward spiking snack foods and drinks with untested herbs. First, it allows manufacturers to pass off soda pop and chips as health foods. In fact, these products should be consumed in moderation, since they're high in calories and usually contain large amounts of sugar (which causes tooth decay) or salt (which may increase the risk of high blood pressure). Furthermore, many of the herbs and other supplements that allegedly make these foods "functional" haven't been well studied. We don't know what effects they have on human health or if they're even safe for daily consumption.

Even functional foods that contain added nutrients we know are valuable, such as calcium and fiber, pose problems. Fiber-enhanced pasta may sound like a great idea, but it shouldn't be consumed at the expense of other important foods. After all, fruits, vegetables, and whole grains provide vitamins, minerals, and micronutrients in addition to healthy doses of fiber. And if you're already getting plenty of fiber in your diet, adding more in the form of a functional food may be a waste of money. The safest bet is to talk to your physician before adding any functional food to your diet.

THE ONE HUNDRED MOST COMMONLY USED HERBS AND SUPPLEMENTS FROM A TO Z

ACIDOPHILUS

Scientific name: *Lactobacillus acidophilus*

What is it?

When most people think of bacteria, they envision armies of microbial nasties that invade our bodies and make us sick. In fact, we need "good" bacteria to keep us healthy, too. *Lactobacillus acidophilus* is one such healthy bacterium. *L. acidophilus* is found in the human digestive system and vagina, where it helps to break down food and keep levels of unhealthy bacteria in check. Good bacteria are sometimes called probiotics.

As a dietary supplement, *L. acidophilus* is often identified simply as acidophilus. It's sold in the form of capsules, liquids, and powders. Yogurt and other fermented dairy products (including some forms of milk) can contain varying levels of *L. acidophilus* and other probiotics.

Why do some people take acidophilus supplements?

To prevent and treat diarrhea and other gastrointestinal problems, vaginal infections, and urinary tract infections. Some people also take acidophilus and other probiotic supplements to lower cholesterol and boost immunity.

Do they work?

Acidophilus is one of the most widely used probiotics, but many other varieties are included in dietary supplements claiming to "support intestinal health." While more study is needed to understand how probiotics work, there is some promising evidence suggesting they may have a role in treating a few specific conditions. For instance, one group of researchers found that an acidophilus preparation (that also contained another strain of probiotic, *Lactobacillus bulgaricus*) appeared to protect patients receiving antibiotic therapy from developing diarrhea, a common side effect. Yet, other studies have found no benefit. Acidophilus was also ineffective in treating traveler's diarrhea in another study, while other probiotics have shown mixed results.

Yogurt has long been a folk remedy for vaginal infections. In a 1995 study, women who ate yogurt that contained acidophilus developed fewer vaginal infections than women who avoided yogurt completely. However, the group of women studied was small and many dropped out when they were asked to stop eating yogurt as part of the experiment. Other studies of probiotics and vaginitis are also flawed, so it's hard to say whether this homemade medicine actually works. Likewise, more research is needed to confirm a role for probiotics in treating urinary tract infections.

Preliminary research suggests that acidophilus may suppress the growth of bacteria that could turn out to play a part in the development of cancers in the digestive tract, but it's a huge stretch to assume that probiotics might prevent cancer. One study of twenty-five people found that eating yogurt containing *L. acidophilus* produced small decreases in cholesterol levels. A larger trial would be needed to draw firm conclusions about a role for these products in preventing heart disease. The theory that probiotics can strengthen the immune system hasn't been adequately studied, either.

What else should I know about acidophilus supplements?

Long-term studies of people who use acidophilus and other probiotics are lacking. Buyer beware: A 1990 analysis of various *Lactobacillus* supplements found that product contamination was common. That doesn't necessarily mean they were unsafe to use, but consumers clearly were not getting the products they paid for.

Most cases of diarrhea, regardless of the cause, are mild and last only a few days. If you're traveling in a developing country, the old advice remains the same: avoid fresh foods and don't drink the water, unless it comes from a sealed bottle.

Bottom line

Early studies suggest that acidophilus may be useful in treating certain types of diarrhea, as well as vaginitis. But more research is needed to prove that these products are safe and effective, so for now acidophilus and other probiotics must be viewed with suspicion. If you have problems with diarrhea or vaginal infections, see a physician.

ALFALFA

Scientific name: *Medicago sativa*
Also known as lucerne, Buffalo grass, Chilean clover, and Purple medick

What is it?

To a farmer, it's cattle feed. To a salad lover, it's a sprout to sprinkle on greens. But alfalfa is also regarded as medicine by some natural healers. The blue-violet flowers and seeds of alfalfa plants are used to make dietary supplements, which are sold as pills, powders, and tinctures.

Why do some people take alfalfa supplements?

It might be easier to list the conditions alfalfa *isn't* used to treat. According to various sources, alfalfa has been used for anemia, arthritis, bladder inflammation, bloating, cholesterol problems, cystitis, diabetes, endometriosis, fever, gout, menopause symptoms, morning sickness, rheumatism, and ulcers. It's also said to "detoxify" the body.

Do they work?

Virtually all medicinal claims made about alfalfa are based on traditional uses and anecdotal evidence. One of the most common folk uses of alfalfa is in the treatment of diabetes, though benefits have only ever been shown in animals. In one small study involving humans (which has not been replicated), people who were given 40 grams of alfalfa seeds at mealtime experienced drops in total and LDL ("bad") cholesterol of up to 26 percent and 30 percent, respectively. But no one should use alfalfa seeds as medicine, since they may have a dark side (see next section). Furthermore, it's hard to find scientific proof that tablets containing dried alfalfa have any therapeutic value. In the words of Varro E. Tyler, author of *The Honest Herbal* and several other books about plant-based medicine, "It is still difficult to understand how alfalfa . . . ever gained a reputation as a medicinal herb."

Fans of alfalfa praise it for being packed with important nutrients, including beta carotene, calcium, magnesium, and potassium, as well as protein. But you can get all those nutrients from a healthy diet.

What else should I know about alfalfa supplements?

Some supplements that contain alfalfa saponins are allegedly "purified" of naturally occurring toxins, though since the Food and Drug Administration doesn't check the quality of dietary supplements, there are no guarantees. Some studies suggest that eating large amounts of alfalfa seeds may cause a dangerous drop in red and white blood cells. Munching raw alfalfa sprouts may not be a good idea, either, for some groups of people in particular. Because alfalfa sprouts have been linked with outbreaks of salmonella food poisoning, the FDA has issued several warnings in the past that children, the elderly, and anyone with a compromised immune system should avoid raw alfalfa sprouts. Likewise, don't consume alfalfa sprouts if you've been prescribed any type of drug intended to suppress the immune system, which can include cyclosporine or any of the corticosteroids.

Bottom line

The medicinal value and safety of alfalfa supplements is unknown. Alfalfa sprouts may be unsafe for certain groups of people.

ALOE VERA

Scientific name: *Aloe barbadensis*

What is it?

This member of the lily family has green, spiky leaves and originally grew in Africa. According to legend, Cleopatra used gel squeezed from the leaves as a skin lotion. Today aloe vera is a ubiquitous ingredient in moisturizers and other cosmetics, as well as sunscreens. You may wonder why this popular skin care ingredient is even mentioned in a book about dietary supplements. In addition to producing the soothing gel, aloe leaves also yield a bitter juice. This juice is dried and sold in powder or capsule form, often blended with other herbs.

Why do some people take aloe vera supplements?

Some proponents of herbal medicine make vague claims about aloe's "healing" properties, but it's best known as a laxative. Likewise, aloe is often included as an ingredient in so-called colon cleansers, which promise to invigorate you by whisking out your gastrointestinal system.

Do they work?

Aloe leaves contain compounds called anthranoids. Scientists believe that these chemicals may act in several ways in the human intestine. First, they decrease the amount of water and electrolytes (such as sodium and potassium) that pass through the intestinal wall and into the bloodstream. Second, anthranoids draw water and electrolytes from the blood and into the intestines. This dual action increases the size of the stool, making aloe a very strong laxative—potentially as strong as a prescription stimulant laxative. So, while we tend to think of aloe as a benign plant, when taken orally it can have serious, druglike side effects (see the next section).

There's no reason to use colon-cleanser products that contain aloe, or any herb, since there's no scientific evidence that they benefit anyone.

What else should I know about aloe vera supplements?

Abuse of aloe vera or any other laxative can cause dehydration and deplete your body of electrolytes, which could lead to serious medical problems. If you take medication to regulate heart rhythm, such as digoxin, loss of potassium could lead to life-threatening complications.

If you have chronic constipation, see a physician. You may feel better simply by adding fiber to your diet, which may have the added benefit of reducing the risk of heart disease and other health problems. But nagging bowel problems can be a symptom of serious medical conditions, such as intestinal obstructions, ulcerative colitis, or appendicitis—many of which require immediate medical attention and may be worsened by the use of a laxative such as aloe.

Finally, constipation is not a one-size-fits-all condition. Some cases respond best to stimulant laxatives, while others need osmotic laxatives such as milk of magnesia (which draw off fluid into the bowel) or stool softeners. Which is all the more reason to talk to your primary-care physician about this uncomfortable problem.

Bottom line

Aloe vera may cause serious side effects, making it a poor choice for self-treating constipation. If you suffer from persistent bowel problems, see a physician.

ALPHA-LIPOIC ACID

Also known as lipoic acid and thiotic acid

What is it?

This naturally occurring compound plays a role in energy metabolism and acts as an antioxidant, meaning that it soaks up and neutralizes damaging free radicals in your system. Alpha-lipoic acid (ALA) supplements are usually sold as capsules.

Why do some people take ALA supplements?

Books touting the benefits of ALA claim that it recharges energy levels and bolsters the body's immune system. Other proponents say that it enhances the activity of antioxidants (such as vitamin E), lowers cholesterol, normalizes blood-sugar levels in diabetics, and prevents cataracts.

Do they work?

The medical use of ALA has primarily been studied for one condition, diabetic neuropathy. The symptoms of diabetic neuropathy can include pain and tingling in the hands and feet. A few German studies have found that large doses of ALA may relieve these symptoms, though one of the trials used an intravenous form of the supplement. More study is necessary to determine whether ALA supplements are a useful treatment for this condition and whether they're as effective as existing medical therapy.

There has been less research to examine other claims that are made about ALA. In one small, preliminary study people with adult-onset diabetes who were given ALA supplements became more sensitive to insulin, which in theory could allow them to use less medication. But the study needs to be replicated with a larger group of subjects. ALA has shown powerful antioxidant activity in test-tube and human studies. In theory, that could mean that ALA supplements might help limit the body's exposure to substances that cause heart disease, cancer, and other conditions. But there is no solid evidence from human studies to support that theory. It's worth noting that several promising antioxidant supplements, such as beta carotene, did not appear to offer any protection from heart disease or cancer when studied in large clinical trials. (Read about antioxidants on page 28).

And speaking of antioxidants: Some laboratory studies suggest that a specific form of ALA may "regenerate" vitamin E, but how that increased antioxidant activity affects human health isn't well understood.

What else should I know about ALA supplements?

The few existing human studies of ALA did not adequately evaluate its safety. Because ALA may alter glucose levels diabetics shouldn't take it or any other dietary supplement without first talking with their physician.

Bottom line

Some studies suggest that ALA may relieve the symptoms of diabetic neuropathy, but more research is needed to prove that it's safe and effective for that purpose. Doctors have at their disposal well-tested medicines for treating pain associated with neuropathy.

AMINO ACID AND PROTEIN SUPPLEMENTS

What are they?

All living matter is made up of large molecules called proteins, which are in turn composed of long chains of smaller units called amino acids. Your body can manufacture many types of amino acids; a well-balanced diet provides the rest. The digestive system breaks down food protein into amino acids, which the body uses to rebuild tissue. Meat, poultry, fish, and dairy products are rich sources of protein. Amino acid and protein dietary supplements are often derived from milk, eggs, or soy, and sold in the form of powdered drink mixes, tablets, capsules, energy bars, or liquids.

Why do some people take amino acid and protein supplements?

To build muscle and strength. Walk into virtually any gym or locker room in the United States and you'll find body builders and athletes who won't go a day without their protein shake or "amino" pills.

Do they work?

If you consume amino acids or proteins in any form, your body uses them to build tissue, including muscle. However, only a small minority of people will benefit from higher-than-normal doses of these nutrients. And it's unclear whether the expensive products sold in health food stores and on the Internet offer any advantage over amino acids and protein found in healthy foods.

Most people get all the protein they need from a typical diet. Even the majority of serious athletes consume plenty of protein, since they have to eat high-calorie diets to compensate for all the energy they burn exercising. But there are a few exceptions. People involved in rigorous strength training (such as body builders and competitive weight lifters) or endurance sports (such as long-distance running) constantly break down muscle tissue. Some research has shown that athletes in these two categories require more protein in their diets than other people, in order to rebuild muscle. According to one formula, these athletes may need up to 1.5 grams per kilogram of body weight per day.

Despite what the ads in fitness magazines may claim, however, there's nothing special about most amino acid and protein formulas, in the opinion of many sports nutritionists. These products provide the same basic building blocks found in high-protein foods, only at a much higher price. Lean meats and poultry, as well as low- or nonfat dairy products, are also excellent sources of protein. Some foods may lack the convenience of a pill or powdered beverage, but meats and milk more than make up for it by offering vitamins and minerals that may be missing in a supplement.

One notable exception to this rule may be dietary supplements containing the amino acid creatine; see page 65.

What else should I know about amino acid and protein supplements?

Some of these products may cause nausea and diarrhea. There is some concern that consuming too much protein can damage the kidneys. At

If you're an endurance athlete or bodybuilder, you may consume protein powders sold in vitamin stores to maintain muscle mass. But you can save money by shopping at your grocery store instead. Depending on the brand you buy, and whether you purchase in bulk, protein supplements cost between 50 cents and $1 per serving, which usually provides approximately 20–25 grams of protein. But you can get the same amount of protein from one cup of dry nonfat milk, mixed with water, for less than 15 cents. Other excellent sources of protein include skinless chicken breast, lean turkey and beef, nonfat yogurt, and soy products.

very high doses, some amino acids may interfere with the body's ability to absorb other amino acids.

Bottom line

Amino acid and protein supplements offer consumers little more than convenience; the safety of using these products in high doses or for extended periods is unknown. Protein-rich foods are cheaper and taste better.

ANTIOXIDANT FORMULAS

What are they?

This may come as a surprise, but there's a downside to breathing. As human cells use the oxygen we take in through respiration, they manufacture toxic waste products known as free radicals. Tobacco smoke, air pollution, radiation, and other sources also expose your body to these unstable molecules, which travel around the body damaging cells. This damage, known as oxidation, can lead to heart disease, cancer, and possibly other diseases. Fortunately, the human body has an elaborate defense system made up of enzymes, vitamins, minerals, and other compounds. These free radical fighters are known collectively as antioxidants.

Fruit, vegetables, and whole grains are the best food sources of antioxidants. Individual vitamins and minerals, such as vitamin C and selenium, are sold as dietary supplements, of course. Antioxidant formulas combine a varied menu of these nutrients in one tablet, capsule, energy bar, or sports drink. Some antioxidant formulas contain doses of vitamins and minerals that far exceed the recommended daily intake. Others may include additional dietary supplements (such as CoQ_{10} or glutathione) or herbal extracts that are known or believed to contain antioxidant compounds.

Why do some people take antioxidant formulas?

These supplements enjoy a reputation for promoting health in various ways. During the last generation antioxidants have been marketed as antiaging potions, which are said to not only fight heart disease and cancer, but also instill youth, maintain vibrant skin, and sharpen the mind. In recent years publishers have released shelves of antioxidant cookbooks and "counters" to help health-minded consumers keep tabs on their intake of these nutrients, in much the same way dieters count calories.

In addition, some bodybuilders take antioxidants on the theory that tough workouts cause large amounts of oxidative damage to the body.

Do they work?

It's impossible to make general statements about antioxidant formulas, since there are so many different combinations of vitamins, minerals, and other compounds packaged together and sold in this category. However, it's fair to say that—despite all the hype—scientists have not been able to prove that high doses of any antioxidant can prevent or cure any disease or health condition. And not for lack of trying, either. Antioxidants represent one of the most intensely studied areas of nutrition. But while a lot has been learned about these nutrients in the last decade or so, much remains unknown.

For instance, lab studies have shown that antioxidants such as vitamin C, vitamin E, beta carotene, and selenium can reduce the activity of free radicals, which can harm blood vessels and promote the growth of tumors. Furthermore, scientists have studied the diet and lifestyle of large populations and learned that people who eat lots of antioxidant-rich fruit and vegetables or take antioxidant vitamin supplements tend to have a low risk for heart disease and cancer.

But these observational studies don't prove cause and effect. The people who remained disease-free may have had other habits, besides healthy diets and vitamin-popping, that protected them. When scientists have conducted tightly controlled experiments, in which subjects who used antioxidant supplements are compared with people given placebos (inactive pills that contain no medicine), the results have been largely disappointing. For instance, test-tube studies show that vitamin E prevents LDL cholesterol from becoming oxidized, which is a necessary step before the fatlike substance clogs arteries. Yet, in controlled trials vitamin E users turn out to be just as likely to have heart attacks and strokes as nonusers. More disturbing is evidence that one widely used antioxidant, beta carotene, may actually increase the risk of lung cancer in smokers.

The final word on these and other antioxidants is far from in, however. It could be, for instance, that higher doses of vitamin E than have been used in clinical trials are needed to prevent cardiovascular disease. Studies of several antioxidants for preventing heart attacks and various cancers are ongoing. Stay tuned, and see separate entries in this book for other antioxidants, including beta carotene, vitamin A, vitamin C, vitamin E, N-acetyl cysteine, alpha-lipoic acid, grape seed extract, pycnogenol, and selenium.

Studies of lab animals suggest that an otherwise healthy person won't live longer simply because he or she takes antioxidant supplements. Frequent, rigorous exercise may increase the activity of free radicals in the body, but there's not enough evidence to suggest that an athlete needs anything more than a balanced diet to get adequate antioxidant protection.

What else should I know about antioxidant formulas?

As mentioned, these preparations may contain very high doses of vitamins and minerals. If you're already taking a multivitamin, adding an antioxidant pill can increase your intake of vitamins and minerals to levels that may cause unwanted side effects.

Many herbs that are sometimes included in antioxidant formulas haven't been adequately studied, so their effects—and potential side effects—are not known.

Bottom line

Antioxidants have been intensely studied, but there's currently no evidence that taking high doses in addition to a balanced diet will confer health benefits. It may be that antioxidant-rich foods contain healthful components not found in supplements. Or that supplements only help people whose bodies lack certain antioxidants. Until conclusive studies are completed, one fact remains clear: You can't lose by eating a healthy diet.

ARGININE

Also known as l-arginine

What is it?

Arginine is one of the amino acids, which are the building blocks of proteins. It plays several critical roles in human health. For example, enzymes in the body convert arginine to nitric oxide, a gas needed to relax the network of vessels that make up the cardiovascular system, allowing for free blood flow. Most humans create adequate amounts of arginine on their own, though it's also present in many foods, particularly meats and dairy products. Arginine supplements are commonly sold as tablets, though other forms, such as candy-bar-like "medical foods" enriched with the amino acid are available, too.

Why do some people take arginine supplements?

To prevent heart disease and improve circulation. Arginine is also promoted as a treatment for erectile dysfunction (or impotence) in men, as well as several other conditions.

Do they work?

Interest in a possible role for arginine in preventing and treating cardiovascular disease and circulatory problems has grown in recent years. In theory, high doses of arginine might dilate, or expand, narrowed blood vessels. That could mean that these supplements would benefit patients with heart failure (inability of the heart to pump adequate amounts of blood, leading to shortness of breath and other symptoms) and angina pectoris (chest pain associated diminished blood flow to the heart muscle).

A few studies have shown that heart failure patients given arginine supplements have improved blood flow and are able to exercise longer. Arginine may also have relieved angina pain in another trial. However, another study failed to show that arginine improved exercise capacity in patients with heart failure, even though it was injected directly into their bodies. What's more, no study has measured whether arginine offers long-lasting cardiovascular benefits. Nor has arginine been compared with standard prescription medications that are known to improve quality of life for patients with heart failure and angina. Although arginine may offer promise, more research is needed to understand how—and how well—it works, and whether it is safe.

The same holds true for the use of arginine to treat other conditions caused by poor circulation, such as intermittent claudication, which causes painful cramps in the legs. There's interesting evidence, but not much (if anything) is known about how arginine stacks up against current medical therapy for this problem. Erectile dysfunction (ED) is often caused by poor blood flow to the penis. Arginine has been touted as a natural alternative to the impotence drug Viagra, but so far studies have been inconclusive.

What else should I know about arginine supplements?

Don't take arginine without the supervision of a physician. It may cause side effects such as headaches and nausea and may interact with some drugs, including oral contraceptives. Also, arbitrarily raising levels of amino acids and nitric oxide may have undesirable health consequences.

Getting arginine by snacking on food bars (as with one widely promoted product) can be expensive and will add calories to your diet.

Bottom line

Arginine has shown promise in early trials of patients with heart failure and other conditions, but more study is needed before this supplement can be recommended as safe or effective. Any measure you take to treat or prevent cardiovascular disease should be guided by a physician.

BARLEY GRASS

Scientific name: *Hordeum vulgare*

What is it?

Barley is a grain grown all over the world, from North Africa to North America. About half the barley harvested is fed to livestock. Of the remaining portion consumed by humans, about 10 percent is malted and used to make beer, as well as whiskey and other distilled beverages.

Barley is a rich source of carbohydrates, and also contains modest amounts of protein, calcium, phosphorus, and lesser quantities of B vitamins and other nutrients. Dietary supplements marketed as barley grass are sold as capsules, powdered beverages, and premixed juice.

Why do some people take barley grass supplements?

Marketers claim that barley grass provides energy and "maintains whole-body health" (according to one Web site). Often referred to as green food, these supplements are said to pack into one capsule or teaspoon of powder all the nutrients you'd get from eating several servings of vegetables. They also contain chlorophyll, the green pigment in plants, of which various claims have been made. Barley grass is also included in so-called detoxifying supplements that allegedly cleanse the body of noxious substances.

Do they work?

Barley is a rich source of fiber, which is known to lower cholesterol, though its effect is modest. A 1994 study found that adding 30 grams of barley flour (mixed in a beverage) to a low-fat diet lowered LDL ("bad") cholesterol by 6.5 percent. However, the researchers didn't take into account other foods the study subjects may have been eating, so it's not clear that the barley was responsible for the improvement in blood-fat levels. And, by the way, 30 grams of bran flour is much more than sellers of barley grass supplements usually recommend to their customers.

Barley flour can also be an effective laxative, as at least one study has shown. That probably explains why it's included in so-called detoxifying supplements, though it's unlikely that these products confer any benefit beyond stimulating bowel movements. Similarly, it's impossible to evaluate a claim such as "maintains whole-body health," since it's vague and meaningless from a medical standpoint. Finally, chlorophyll has been studied for its potential role as a cancer fighter, but there's no solid evidence that it confers any significant health benefits.

What else should I know about barley grass supplements?

No major side effects have been reported in the few existing studies of barley grass, though the safety of these supplements hasn't been formally researched.

Bottom line

The American Heart Association and the American Cancer Society recommend consuming lots of fiber—in the form of food, not supplements. If you're taking barley grass pills or powders (or any other dietary supplement) to get a dose of fiber, you may be missing out on other nutrients found in fruit, vegetables, and whole grains.

BEE POLLEN

What is it?

The fine powder produced by flowers as fertilizer, and that causes people with allergies to dread spring. Some pollen sold in supplement form (usually as tablets) is gathered by placing a specially designed portal at the entrance of a hive, which brushes the powder from bees' legs. However, *bee pollen* is occasionally a misnomer, since some commercial preparations contain pollen that's harvested by humans.

Why do some people take bee pollen supplements?

Bee pollen is often called the perfect food and has long been used for a variety of purposes by traditional healers. Today, some athletes take bee pollen supplements to gain strength, speed, and durability. Off the playing field, bee pollen has a reputation for helping to fight physical and mental fatigue. Herbalists sometimes recommend bee pollen to men suffering from prostatitis and enlarged prostate.

Do they work?

Despite the buzz about bee pollen among athletes, there's little reason to believe that it will make you speedier or stronger. A British study in the early 1980s found that well-trained teenage swimmers who took pollen tablets performed no better or worse than other swimmers given placebo pills. However, it's not possible to draw conclusions from this study, since it involved just a few athletes. Germany's Commission E says pollen acts as a "roborant for feebleness," meaning it restores strength and vigor. But there's little scientific evidence to back up such a claim.

A few small, preliminary studies suggest that bee pollen supplements may provide mild relief from the annoying symptoms of an enlarged prostate, but the findings need to be confirmed with a well-designed experiment in a larger group of patients. Articles in medical journals dating back to the 1960s mention pollen as a potential cure for prostatitis (a painful inflammation), but no scientist has proven that it works.

What else should I know about bee pollen supplements?

If you're allergic to pollen, stay away from these supplements.

Bee pollen contains vitamin C and other nutrients, but it's questionable whether that makes it a "perfect food." A balanced diet provides all the zip most people need to compete in recreational sports or get through a day at the office. The herb saw palmetto (see page 171) and the drug finasteride probably do a better job of treating noncancerous prostate enlargement, though the symptoms of this condition should be evaluated by a physician.

Bottom line

They may have a certain exotic allure, but bee pollen supplements lack evidence to recommend their use. Men who experience pain or difficulty in urinating should see a physician.

BETA CAROTENE

What is it?

Carotenoids are pigments found in many plant foods. Mammals, including humans, can convert carotenoids to vitamin A, which is needed to protect cells and promote healthy eyes and skin (and whose role in human health is discussed in a separate entry—see page 189). The carotenoids—particularly beta carotene—may play other important roles in safeguarding human health. For example, beta carotene is a potent antioxidant, meaning that it scavenges naturally occurring molecules known as free radicals from the body.

Brilliantly colored fruits and vegetables, such as carrots, leafy greens, red peppers, sweet potatoes, and apricots, are good sources of beta carotene. As a dietary supplement, beta carotene is usually sold as a pill or capsule.

Why do some people take beta carotene supplements?

Many people bank on beta carotene's antioxidant powers as a way to prevent cancer and cardiovascular disease.

Do they work?

Intense interest in beta carotene's disease-fighting potential was heightened with the publication of research revealing that people who eat lots of vegetables that are rich in this nutrient have a low risk for cancer and heart disease. However, subsequent studies to determine whether taking beta carotene supplements can prevent either of these diseases have yielded conflicting and often unimpressive results.

Consider what happened when scientists studied over twenty-nine thousand male smokers in Finland to see if beta carotene can prevent lung cancer. The men were split into four groups. Some were given daily supplements of beta carotene, some received vitamin E, and a third group got both. The final group was given inactive placebo pills. The men took the supplements each day for at least five years. The research team came to a surprising conclusion at the study's end: Not only did beta carotene fail to protect the men from lung cancer, but it appeared to make them *more* likely to develop the disease.

Was the Finnish study a fluke? A second scientific paper, published two years later, suggests that it may not have been. This time smokers, ex-smokers, and asbestos workers were given a combination of beta carotene and vitamin A (in the form of retinol). And once again beta carotene appeared to worsen the risk for lung cancer.

Further studies of people taking beta carotene suggest that it does not prevent other types of cancer. However, one important trial demonstrated that retinoic acid—a form of vitamin A, which is produced from beta carotene—decreased the risk of recurrent tumors in patients who had been treated for cancer of the head and neck. Given these varied results, it's clear that more study is needed to understand whether beta carotene or some other form of vitamin A has a role in cancer prevention.

The two studies described above also investigated whether beta carotene prevented cardiovascular disease, with similar results. In the first study, men who took beta carotene were slightly more likely than men taking sugar pills to die of heart disease. The second trial found no heart benefit to taking beta carotene and retinol. Furthermore, at least one other large study determined that beta carotene supplements don't protect against fatal heart attacks, while another found that they caused a slight increase in the incidence of angina pectoris (chest pain caused by diminished blood supply to the heart).

What else should I know about beta carotene supplements?

In the amount of research described above, limited beta carotene appears to be safe; the body only converts as much as it needs into vitamin A. (High doses of vitamin A supplements, meanwhile, can be toxic.)

Beta carotene may cause the skin to turn orange.

Bottom line

Most studies have shown that beta carotene supplements do not prevent cancer; some research suggests that they may even be harmful to some people. There's also no evidence that high doses of beta carotene will prevent heart attacks. A sound diet probably provides all the beta carotene and other antioxidants necessary to maintain good health.

BILBERRY

Scientific name: *Vaccinium myrtillus*
Also known by many other names, including huckleberry, whortleberry, and European blueberry
Not to be confused with bog bilberry

What is it?

A relative of the blueberry plant, this hardy shrub grows in northern Europe and North America. The berries are dried to produce an extract that's usually sold in the form of capsules and tablets. Don't use bilberry leaves (see below).

Why do some people take bilberry supplements?

During World War II, British fighter pilots reportedly ate bilberry jam before heading out on night missions, believing that something in the berries helped their eyes adjust to the dark faster. That belief has persisted, and today bilberry supplements are popular with people who want to improve their night vision. In fact, bilberry is sometimes called the vision herb, since it's also recommended by herbalists to treat several eye diseases, including cataracts, macular degeneration, and retinopathy, a condition that afflicts some diabetics.

Furthermore, bilberry is used for several other conditions, from the mundane (diarrhea) to the serious (heart disease).

Do they work?

The evidence that bilberry supplements clear up night blindness is blurry, indeed. Believers point out that bilberries contain compounds called anthocyanosides, which may play a role in regenerating purple pigment in the eye that's critical to seeing in the dark. However, in the late '90s researchers in Israel staged two experiments to determine whether taking supplements that contain anthocyanosides improves night vision. Neither attempt revealed any benefit. Men who took the supplements were tested against others given fake pills in a lab designed to measure night vision. Unfortunately, one group remained just as much in the dark as the other.

The young men in these two studies were healthy and had no reported problems with night vision. It's possible that subjects who actually suffer from nyctalopia, or night blindness, might be helped by taking bilberry or some other supplement that contains anthocyanosides. But more studies are needed to confirm that theory.

A very modest amount of research suggests that bilberry extract may benefit other, more serious eye conditions, including cataracts and diabetic retinopathy. But no study has ever shown that taking these supplements prevents blindness of any kind. Bilberry's therapeutic value in preventing or treating other conditions is largely unknown. However, dried bilberries (but not fresh) are rich in tannins, which means they might help clear up a case of diarrhea (though this use hasn't been adequately studied).

What else should I know about bilberry supplements?

Not much is known about long-term use of bilberry supplements. Don't eat fresh bilberries if you're battling diarrhea; they could make the problem worse. Talk to your doctor instead.

Avoid supplements that contain bilberry leaves; German health authorities give them a thumbs down, since at high doses they may cause a long list of health problems, including anemia, jaundice, loss of muscle, and others.

Bottom line

This berry may produce a tasty jam, but it does not appear to improve vision, according to a limited number of studies. Other health benefits associated with bilberry should be regarded with caution, as they're unproven.

BIOTIN

What is it?

Biotin is one of the B vitamins. One important role for this nutrient is to help the body use carbohydrates and fats from food. Biotin is present pretty much wherever the other B vitamins are found, which includes many plant and animal foods. What's more, microorganisms in your gut produce the vitamin, too. The average American consumes 150–300 micrograms of biotin every day. Biotin supplements are usually sold as tablets.

Why do some people take biotin supplements?

If you own a horse, you may feed biotin to old Nelly for stronger hooves. Like hooves, human toe- and fingernails are made of a tough substance called keratin, which is why some people take biotin to treat brittle nails. For some reason, these sorts of nail problems are more common in women than in men. Biotin supplements are also said to promote lustrous hair and healthy skin.

Do they work?

Biotin deficiency is rare, but can lead to hair loss and skin problems. There's simply no scientific evidence, however, that consuming mega doses of this B vitamin will make the hair and skin of a healthy person look any better. A few small investigations have probed the suggestion that biotin supplements can cure brittle nails. A study involving thirty-five patients at a clinic in New York City found that two-thirds had firmer, smoother nails after taking biotin supplements for a few months. Several earlier European studies came up with similar results. However, even the authors of the New York City study concluded that biotin's value in treating this cosmetic problem needs to be validated with a larger trial.

What else should I know about biotin supplements?

There's no established recommended daily intake for biotin, though it appears to be safe in large doses. Still, adequate safety studies on these supplements haven't been conducted, so talk to a physician before taking them for stronger nails or any reason. And by all means, if you do have brittle nails, schedule an office visit soon. The problem can be associated with several potentially serious medical conditions.

Bottom line

Biotin is present in so many foods that deficiency is extremely rare. It's not clear whether these supplements can strengthen brittle nails. This condition should be examined by a physician.

BLACK COHOSH

Scientific name: *Cimicifuga racemosa*
Not be confused with blue cohosh

What is it?

Black cohosh is a plant that grows wild throughout the east coast of the United States and Canada; it's related to the buttercup. Native Americans boiled the roots and stems of black cohosh to make a medicinal tea, which was used to treat everything from sore throats to snake bites.

Black cohosh was also an ingredient in a popular elixir sold in this country during the late nineteenth century, known as Lydia Pinkham's Vegetable Compound (in which the main ingredient was alcohol). Today, you'll usually find black cohosh sold in capsule form, though liquid extract and teas are available, too.

Why do some people take black cohosh supplements?

Herbalists still recommend black cohosh for a variety of ailments, including bad coughs. But it's best known as a kind of superherb for women, particularly at midlife. When a woman reaches menopause, her production of estrogen drops dramatically. This hormonal change can produce a variety of symptoms, including hot flashes and night sweats (which plague about three-quarters of postmenopausal women). These symptoms can be relieved by hormone-replacement therapy, but many women can't or won't take HRT. Instead, some turn to black cohosh and other herbs to chill out. This herb is also used to take the edge off PMS (premenstrual syndrome) and ease the pain of menstrual cramps.

Do they work?

Some research, much of it performed in Germany, suggests that black cohosh helps diminish the symptoms associated with menopause, possibly because it contains compounds that act like estrogen. However, many doctors in this country would like to see more proof. Several trials have shown that women had fewer symptoms related to menopause while consuming black cohosh. But these studies have involved too few women to draw firm conclusions or had some critical flaw that makes their findings questionable. One trial involving 85 breast cancer patients—half received black cohosh, while the others were given placebos—found that the herb offered no relief to women experiencing postmenopausal symptoms. More study is necessary to learn more about who, if anyone, benefits from using black cohosh.

The German government has approved the use of black cohosh for PMS and menstrual cramps, though there's little scientific evidence that it works.

What else should I know about black cohosh supplements?

The existing studies on black cohosh have not adequately assessed its safety. However, taking too much is known to cause nausea and other stomach complaints. Pregnant women should not use this herb; there is some concern that it may increase the risk of spontaneous abortion. Black cohosh may interfere with the body's ability to absorb iron. (Black cohosh is unrelated to blue cohosh, which should probably be avoided altogether, especially if you're pregnant. The latter herb may induce labor.) There isn't much information about long-term use of black cohosh, which is why German health officials discourage use of the herb for longer than six months.

As mentioned above, black cohosh may contain substances that act like estrogen. Levels of this hormone are diminished in women after they reach menopause. Replacing estrogen with prescription hormones not only controls symptoms of menopause, but is also known to help prevent osteoporosis and decrease a woman's risk for cardiovascular disease. No one knows whether black cohosh provides these same benefits. Furthermore, estrogen may increase the risk of uterine and breast cancer. Women who have an intact uterus who take prescription hormone replacement are given progesterone to reduce the increased risk of uterine cancer that accompanies the use of estrogen. (Progesterone may also decrease the risk of ovarian cancer.) No one knows whether black cohosh increases the chances of developing uterine cancer or breast cancer; if it does, women who rely on it to treat hot flashes and other symptoms of menopause without the protection of progesterone may be unwittingly increasing their disease risk.

Bottom line

Until further studies on black cohosh are completed, it's not clear whether this herb offers a safe and effective way to relieve hot flashes and other symptoms of menopause. Any woman who has reached menopause should discuss hormone-replacement therapy with her physician.

CALCIUM

What is it?

Calcium is the building block of bone and teeth, though a very small amount you consume also plays a role in nerve transmission, muscle contraction, and other body functions. This mineral is found in many common foods, particularly dairy products. Calcium tablets outsell all but a few dietary supplements in the United States. You'll find the mineral in just about any multivitamin, too, and many antacid pills contain calcium.

Why do some people take calcium supplements?

To prevent osteoporosis, the fragile bone disease that afflicts about 10 million Americans and can be blamed for 1.5 million fractures each year. About seventy-five thousand people in this country die each year from complications related to broken hips alone. Osteoporosis isn't just a concern for women, either; by age seventy-five, about one-third of all men are affected by the disease.

Do they work?

There's no question that calcium is critical to bone health, and studies show that supplements can help fill the void if you don't get enough from your diet (and many Americans don't). In one study, a group of women who had reached menopause was assembled. On average, the women consumed about 750 milligrams of calcium per day. Half were given daily supplements of 1,000 milligrams of the mineral, while the other half received sugar pills. After two years researchers determined that the women taking calcium had slowed bone loss. Another study found that elderly women were less likely to suffer broken bones if they consumed calcium with vitamin D.

In recent years scientists have realized that a diet rich in calcium may have added health benefits. In particular, a 1999 study found that calcium supplements may play a role in preventing colon cancer. The study involved women who had had polyps removed from their colons. Polyps are benign growths that can turn cancerous. Taking a supplement containing 1,200 milligrams of calcium every day for a few years appeared to cut the women's risk of polyp recurrence. But while this study showed a modest benefit, further research is needed to confirm the link between calcium and this often-deadly cancer.

What else should I know about calcium supplements?

When taken at the recommended daily allowance, calcium supplements are safe for most people, though in some cases they may cause gas or constipation. When possible, take calcium supplements with food, to make sure that they're fully absorbed by your body. Government guidelines suggest that men and women under fifty get at least 1,000 milligrams of calcium per day; people over fifty should consume at least 1,200 milligrams. Avoid superhigh doses, which may block the absorption of other minerals and can even be toxic, especially when taken with high levels of vitamin D.

An analysis published in the *Journal of the American Medical Association* found that several popular brands of calcium supplements contained lead. Reports such as this may be a good argument for sticking with established manufacturers when you shop for these products.

A healthy diet can provide all or most of the calcium you need. Remember, dietary supplements are not a substitute for a healthy diet, which can decrease your risk of obesity, heart disease, and cancer. To get your dose of calcium from your diet, consume lots of low- or nonfat dairy products, vegetables with dark green leaves (such as spinach and broccoli), canned fish with bones (such as sardines), legumes, and calcium-fortified products, such as orange juice.

Bottom line

There's much more to preventing osteoporosis than taking calcium pills. Talk to your physician about a healthy diet, exercise, vitamin D, the use of supplemental estrogen (for women past menopause), new medications, *and* calcium supplements.

CARNITINE

Also known as l-carnitine

What is it?

Carnitine is a vitamin-like substance that carries fat into cells, where it can be metabolized as energy. It's found in muscle, including the tissue that forms heart muscle. Meat and dairy products are good sources of carnitine, though your body can produce its own. As a dietary supplement, carnitine is sold as capsules, and tablets, and in liquid form.

Why do some people take carnitine supplements?

To improve athletic performance, build muscle, and lose weight. There's also growing interest in claims that carnitine may benefit some forms of heart disease, as well as Alzheimer's disease.

Do they work?

According to locker-room wisdom, carnitine supplements give you more energy to exercise and trim pounds simply by making it easier for your body to burn fat. In theory, if you're stoked up on carnitine, your muscles will rely on fat as its preferred energy source during a workout. That way you save carbohydrates to burn later on, giving you greater endurance to exercise longer. Athletes and supplement sellers also claim that carnitine levels are exhausted by exercise, suggesting that supplements can provide an added boost. But none of these theories has been proven. Studies of athletes who use carnitine have produced contradictory results. In fact, experiments with swimmers and distance runners failed to show any competitive advantage to taking carnitine supplements. Other research shows that a hard workout does *not* deplete the body of carnitine. This supplement may be a staple in the gym and weight room, but more studies are needed to determine whether all those athletes and bodybuilders should save their money.

That goes for dieters, too. The theory that carnitine tells your body to burn the fat on your waistline and hips may be alluring, but it's not backed by scientific evidence. In fact, one small study in Australia found that the supplements didn't help moderately obese women shed pounds.

A modest amount of research, mostly performed overseas, has found that patients with certain heart conditions have improved after taking carnitine supplements. For example, several studies suggest that the symptoms of angina pectoris (chest pain during physical exertion that's caused by too little blood flowing to the heart) may be improved in patients given carnitine. Preliminary research also hints that the supplement may prolong survival among patients with heart failure. However, much more research is needed, and these uses of carnitine are still considered experimental.

Preliminary research has been conducted on patients with Alzheimer's disease using altered forms of carnitine, but the results are not conclusive and no one should take supplements to prevent or treat this serious condition.

What else should I know about carnitine supplements?

Gastrointestinal complaints such as diarrhea and vomiting are among the most common side effects associated with carnitine. The supplements may also cause high blood pressure, dizziness, and some other symptoms. People diagnosed with seizure disorders should use particularly great caution.

Bottom line

There is no solid evidence that carnitine supplements build muscle or burn fat. Some promising research suggests that carnitine may benefit patients with existing heart disease, but more study is needed to understand its effects and safety.

CAT'S CLAW

Scientific name: *Uncaria tomentosa*
Also known as *uña de gato*

What is it?

This woody vine grows in the rain forests of South America, where it's an important plant in the medicine practiced by various Indian tribes. Rain forest Indians use cat's claw as an all-around health tonic and to treat specific conditions, including upset stomach, fever, and even some cancers. Traditional healers boil the bark to make a tea, but the herb is widely available in the form of tablets, capsules, and liquid extract.

Why do some people take cat's claw supplements?

Modern herbalists recommend it for a variety of conditions, in particular arthritis, high blood pressure, and digestive disorders, including diverticulitis, ulcers, and hemorrhoids. Some people who are HIV positive or have AIDS take cat's claw to supplement a regimen of AZT.

Do they work?

There is some laboratory evidence suggesting that compounds found in cat's claw may relieve inflammation, strengthen the immune system, and fight the growth of malignant tumors. But so far most studies have been limited to test tubes and lab animals, so it's impossible to say whether the herb would help treat or prevent arthritis, AIDS, cancer, or any other disease in humans. Furthermore, no adequate study has been performed to determine whether cat's claw is any better than prescription and over-the-counter drugs for treating gastrointestinal problems.

What else should I know about cat's claw supplements?

There are few, if any, reports of adverse reactions to cat's claw. However, it's impossible to determine whether any dosage of this herb is truly safe, since its toxicity hasn't been adequately tested.

Bottom line

Scientists have barely studied cat's claw; no one knows whether it's safe or effective for treating any condition.

CAYENNE

Scientific name: *Capsicum frutescens* and others

What is it?

You probably know this incendiary powder as a spice. But cayenne pepper, produced from dried red chilies, has been used as medicine since the days of the ancient Mayans. Chilies contain a substance called capsaicin that not only makes them hot, but also has gained attention in recent years for its potential therapeutic value. Prescription and over-the-counter drugs that contain capsaicin, in the form of skin creams and gels, are available. As a dietary supplement, cayenne is usually sold in capsules.

Why do some people take cayenne supplements?

The pepper-packed pills are used for a variety of purposes, among them relieving pain and indigestion. They're used to ward off colds and sore throats, too. Cayenne is also often included in herbal preparations bearing claims such as "supports cardiovascular health."

Do they work?

Creams and gels containing capsaicin have been approved by the Food and Drug Administration for the treatment of pain associated with arthritis and certain other conditions. Though it stings at first, topical capsaicin appears to desensitize pain receptors. Because these products are classified as over-the-counter drugs, you can be sure they've undergone testing to prove that they're effective.

But that's not the case for capsules or any other oral form of cayenne sold in health food stores. Like the other dietary supplements described in this book, they don't require FDA approval before being sold. And the simple fact is that most of the claims made about oral cayenne supplements that appear in herb guides and on the Internet are not supported by solid evidence. Few studies have examined the oral use of capsaicin as medicine, and most of those have been performed in test tubes or in animals. In one of the few human studies to examine the health benefits of capsaicin, consuming chili peppers appeared to offer some protection against aspirin, which can damage the lining of the stomach. However, more research is needed to understand capsaicin's role in safeguarding the stomach from ulcers and other injuries. And there's no solid evidence that capsaicin supplements reduce the risk of heart disease or ease the pain of arthritis.

What else should I know about cayenne supplements?

The risks associated with eating fresh or cooked chilies are well known: a burning sensation on the lips and tongue, perspiration, even tears. Some side effects that have been associated with use of the capsules include heartburn, kidney and liver damage, and other serious side effects. Laboratory studies suggest that capsaicin may even promote cancer.

Consult a physician before using capsaicin cream on your skin; it has reportedly caused allergic reactions, skin rashes, and blisters. Do not apply the cream on or near the eyes.

Bottom line

The medical use of cayenne pepper in capsule form hasn't been well studied and may be dangerous. Applied topically, the drug capsaicin in cayenne may help provide pain relief, but may also have serious side effects; use it only under the supervision of a physician.

Researchers at Yale found that chewing taffy made with capsaicin provided brief, modest pain relief for cancer patients with mouth sores caused by chemotherapy.

CHAMOMILE

Scientific name: *Matricaria recutita**
Also known as camomile

What is it?

This daisy look-alike (the two plants belong to the same family) grows wild and is cultivated in the United States and Europe. The flower heads are dried before being used as medicine. Chamomile is perhaps most commonly prepared as a tea (though brewing reduces the level of active ingredients). Until recently it was hard to find chamomile capsules in this country, but they're now widely available. The dried leaves are also steamed to extract a blue essential oil from the flowers.

Why do some people use chamomile supplements?

If you're visiting relatives in Berlin and develop an upset stomach, your hosts may brew you a cup of chamomile tea instead of offering an Alka-Seltzer. Cut your finger? Out comes the chamomile again, this time moistened and applied directly to the wound, to make it heal faster and kill bacteria. According to the German government, chamomile can also be used to treat inflammation (including hemorrhoids) and fever, quell stomach cramps, and even prevent body odor.

In this country, chamomile is largely thought of as a sleep aid and stress buster. Many herbal preparations that promise to help you relax contain chamomile, along with other herbs.

* There are several related plants that go by the name chamomile; we'll only discuss German chamomile here, since it's the variety most often sold in the United States.

Do they work?

According to anecdote, taking chamomile in some form before going to bed does speed up the trip to la-la land. But no conclusive scientific trials have been performed to prove whether it works better than a placebo, or even a mug of warm milk. Still, if caffeine keeps you up at night, a cup of chamomile tea—which does not contain the stimulant—makes a better after-dinner drink than coffee or regular tea.

As for stress, simply stopping to sip a cup of tea may be enough to mellow out a set of ragged nerves. According to some research, a compound in chamomile called apigenin may act on the brain in a way similar to benzodiazepines, which are drugs commonly prescribed to treat anxiety. However, the folk wisdom that chamomile eases anxiety in humans has not been confirmed in human studies.

As for chamomile's gut-soothing, wound-healing, skin-clearing qualities: the evidence is largely anecdotal, though some lab studies suggest that apigenin and other compounds in chamomile may reduce inflammation and destroy bacteria. However, in one study a mouthwash made from chamomile failed to prevent mouth sores from chemotherapy in cancer patients.

What else should I know about chamomile supplements?

As an herb, chamomile is generally considered nontoxic, with one or two exceptions. If you're allergic to chrysanthemums, ragweed, or any other member of the daisy family, exposure to chamomile could cause skin rash and, according to some reports, anaphylactic shock. Pregnant women should not use chamomile, since very large doses reportedly cause miscarriages. The safety of chamomile supplements hasn't been studied, though it's believed that high levels of this herb may interfere with the body's ability to absorb iron.

If chamomile comes in contact with bare skin it may cause a rash. Because this herb may contain potent chemicals, it could be unwise to use chamomile if you're taking blood thinning or sedative medications. Consuming alcohol may be unadvisable, too.

Bottom line

Many people find a cup of chamomile tea to be soothing, but there's not much evidence that taking this herb in pill form will ease anxiety or make you sleepy. If you feel chronically stressed out, struggle with frequent insomnia, or your stomach is always in knots, talk to your primary-care physician; these symptoms may be signs of more serious conditions.

CHILDREN'S VITAMINS

What are they?

Multivitamins that may be chewable, fruit-flavored, or shaped like cartoon characters. These supplements contain a blend of nutrients that's designed to help a child meet or exceed the recommended daily intake for vitamins and minerals. Some varieties also include medicinal herbs. Children's multivitamins are very popular in the United States. Over half of all preschool children take them, though older kids are less likely to receive these once-a-day pills.

Children's multivitamins are usually sold as liquid drops for the very young (under two or three years) and as tablets for older children.

Why do some people give their children vitamin supplements?

To make sure their children receive adequate nutrition.

Do they work?

Most experts believe that children—like adults—should rely on food as their source of nutrients. The American Academy of Pediatrics, for instance, doesn't recommend giving vitamin supplements to children. (One exception: Parents of families that live in parts of the country with unfluoridated drinking water should ask their physician whether they and their children should use fluoride supplements.) When you consider that scientists are constantly discovering new, health-promoting micronutrients in foods, which are *not* found in multivitamins, it's a tough argument to counter.

That is, unless you're the parent of a finicky child. In fact, some nutritionists and doctors in this country recognize that it's often difficult to convince a child to eat enough of the right foods, so they may recommend giving infants and children multivitamins as insurance. If your child is otherwise healthy, talk to his or her pediatrician about the merits of multivitamins.

For some kids, however, vitamin supplements may be essential, including children who:

> have been diagnosed with a chronic disease or anorexia
> have poor appetites or eating habits
> are vegetarians

What's more, teenage girls who have heavy menstrual periods may require additional iron to avoid becoming anemic. If you think your child may have special dietary requirements, talk to a physician. Addressing your child's nutritional needs may not be as simple as giving him or her a multivitamin.

What else should I know about children's vitamins?

Although multivitamins in general are considered very safe, they should still be administered by parents. In large amounts, some vitamins and minerals can be toxic, so don't exceed the recommended dosage. And it may be unsafe to give a child any supplement containing medicinal herbs. Many have not been adequately tested, so there's no way to know if they're safe.

Bottom line

Don't assume your child needs a multivitamin; talk over his or her nutritional needs with a physician.

CHITOSAN

What is it?

When food processors prepare shrimp, crab, or lobster meat for canning or freezing, they don't throw out the leftover shells. These outer skeletons are valued for their high content of chitin, a substance found in certain other animals (particularly insects) and plants that has a number of industrial applications. One is to absorb grease and oil in the treatment of wastewater. Chitosan is derived from chitin and sold as a dietary supplement in capsule or tablet form.

Why do some people take chitosan supplements?

To take the pain out of weight loss. Companies that sell chitosan frequently claim it's a "fat blocker" that allows you to lose weight while eating decadent foods. Chitosan is also sometimes referred to as marine fiber and used to lower cholesterol.

Do they work?

Like fiber, chitosan can't be digested by humans. It's also believed that chitosan binds with lipids, such as fat molecules, which prevents them from being absorbed through the intestinal tract. Rats given chitosan excrete large amounts of fat. Some unconfirmed preliminary research suggests that people who consume low-calorie diets may increase their weight loss by taking chitosan.

However, infomercials and other ads for this supplement suggest that you can eat as much junk food as you like and still shed pounds if you take chitosan. In 1999 a group of British researchers set out to determine whether that's true. They gave chitosan to one group of overweight people and empty placebo pills to another. Both groups were sent home with orders to eat their normal diets. A month later neither group had lost weight. This small study involved just thirty people and would need to be repeated to better understand chitosan's value (or lack thereof) as a weight loss aid. More important, chitosan should be compared with safe, established methods of weight loss, particularly prescription drugs (such as orlistat) that also act by blocking the absorption of fat.

Similarly, chitosan's usefulness in lowering cholesterol has only been measured in a few studies. It may prove to offer some benefits, but should first be compared with existing medications that are known to lower cholesterol.

What else should I know about chitosan supplements?

No one who is allergic to seafood should use chitosan. If these supplements actually block the absorption of fats, then they may cause oily stools. Chitosan may also interfere with the body's ability to absorb certain vitamins, known as fat-soluble vitamins; that is, if there's no fat in the gut, these vitamins don't dissolve and simply wash out of the system.

Bottom line

Chitosan has not been adequately tested as a weight-loss aid, so no one can say whether it's safe and effective. Instead of using untested products, speak with a physician about proven methods for shedding pounds.

CHOLINE

What is it?

Choline is a vitamin-like nutrient that's a component of many important molecules in the body. One of them is the chemical acetylcholine, which is needed for transmitting nerve impulses. (Another is lecithin, or phosphatidylcholine [see page 124]). Rich sources of choline include egg yolks, liver and other organ meats, nuts, wheat germ, soybeans, and spinach. Choline supplements are sold as liquids, capsules, powders, and granules (which are sprinkled on food or dissolved in beverages).

Why do some people take choline supplements?

To protect the brain and liver, as well as lower cholesterol. Also, some athletes use choline in the belief that it improves aerobic endurance.

Do they work?

Much of the research on this substance has involved its chemical fore-runner, lecithin (see page 124), which most people find easier to tolerate. People with Alzheimer's disease may have below-normal levels of choline in their brains, according to postmortem studies. However, there's no way of knowing whether choline supplements protect against this disease, since their use for that purpose hasn't been adequately studied.

Acetylcholine is necessary for muscle contraction. Studies have shown that choline levels may drop during intense physical exercise. These two concepts have led some sports physiologists to surmise that loading up on choline before a bout of training may increase an athlete's endurance. But in several studies involving cyclists and soldiers exercising on treadmills, choline supplements failed to increase physical endurance.

There's no solid evidence that increasing choline levels beyond that supplied by a normal diet will lower cholesterol or protect the liver from cirrhosis, hepatitis, or other conditions.

What else should I know about choline supplements?

Like many supplements, choline may cause stomach upset and diarrhea, especially in large doses. But choline's biggest drawback is that it can give your breath a fishy odor. Little is known about long-term use of these supplements.

Bottom line

There's no conclusive evidence that choline supplements protect brain functioning or boost endurance.

CHONDROITIN

Pronounced "con-DROYT-in"
Usually sold as chondroitin sulfate

What is it?

Chondroitin is a substance found in various types of body tissue, including cartilage, the smooth tissue that lines the surface of joints. It's sometimes called the liquid magnet, because it draws fluid into cartilage, making it more elastic. It also stifles the activity of enzymes that can damage cartilage. Chondroitin supplements are produced synthetically, but are also extracted from shark and bovine (as in cows and oxen) cartilage. They're sold as capsules and tablets, often combined with glucosamine.

Why do some people use chondroitin supplements?

With age, cartilage produces less chondroitin, which contributes to the pain and stiffness of osteoarthritis, a disease that afflicts over 40 million Americans. Chondroitin supplements are designed to restore elasticity to cartilage. Chondroitin became popular in the United States after the publication of several books, including *The Arthritis Cure*, which extolled the benefits of the supplement, particularly when taken with glucosamine (see page 105).

Do they work?

According to a review of fifteen studies published in the *Journal of the American Medical Association*, chondroitin may provide modest relief from arthritis pain and discomfort. (The same analysis found similar benefits for glucosamine.) Another review, in the *Journal of Rheumatology*, looked at seven studies comparing chondroitin supplements to placebo. The authors found that arthritis sufferers who got the real pills experienced a 50 percent improvement in symptoms. However, the authors of both studies say more research is needed to confirm chondroitin's role as a dependable treatment for osteoarthritis.

What else should I know about chondroitin supplements?

These supplements are generally considered risk-free, though more studies are needed to determine whether it's safe to use chondroitin for long periods. Most studies suggest that you may need to take chondroitin for several months before feeling any pain relief.

If you've considered trying chondroitin because you fear side effects associated with drugs, it's important to know that prescription medications known as COX-2 inhibitors treat joint pain, but are less likely than older drugs to cause gastrointestinal side effects.

If you have recurrent joint pain, see a physician. The pain may not be from osteoarthritis; aching bones can also be caused by other disorders, such as rheumatoid arthritis (which occurs when the body's immune system literally attacks its own tissue) that require a doctor's attention.

Bottom line

Chondroitin may be an effective treatment for osteoarthritis. However, further studies are needed to reveal how it works and whether it's safe to use for long periods. Don't self-treat chronic joint pain; see a physician, who can determine the cause of the problem and develop a treatment plan that best suits your needs.

CHROMIUM

What is it?

Chromium is an essential trace mineral, which means your body needs it to run properly, but only in small amounts. In the laboratory, chromium appears to enhance the effect of the hormone insulin, which helps nutrients enter cells to be used as energy. This mineral occurs in tiny concentrations in some foods, including organ meats, broccoli, whole grains, nuts, and brewer's yeast. Chromium supplements are sold as capsules and tablets, usually in the form of chromium picolinate or chromium nicotinate.

Why do some people take chromium supplements?

Most consumers who use chromium undoubtedly believe it will reshape their bodies—either help them shed pounds or pack on muscle. Some people with adult-onset diabetes use chromium supplements to control blood sugar. Likewise, chromium is also sometimes used to lower cholesterol.

Do they work?

Chromium believers say the mineral creates shapelier bodies by making cells burn nutrients and store muscle-building amino acids more efficiently. Athletes in particular get a hard sell for this supplement, since some research suggests that exercise increases the loss of chromium, leading to the idea that athletes may be deficient in the mineral.

In fact, documented cases of chromium deficiency are uncommon in the United States. And evidence that supplements of the mineral increase weight loss or build muscle is at best contradictory. Much-hyped studies in the 1980s suggested that chromium picolinate acts like anabolic steroids; college athletes who used the supplements were said to have become leaner and more muscular. However, those studies have been criticized for using an imprecise method of measuring muscle and body fat. Several subsequent studies, using more advanced methods of measuring body composition, have failed to confirm chromium picolinate's reputation as a fat-burning, muscle-making supplement. Studies show that many people who increase the amount of chromium in their diets end up eliminating most of it in their urine.

The role of chromium supplements for controlling blood sugar in diabetics remains controversial. Some studies offer promise that they might help, while others haven't shown a consistent benefit. The American Diabetes Association does not recommend the use of supplemental chromium. Chromium hasn't been adequately studied for lowering cholesterol and other blood lipids. Furthermore, no one should attempt to alter his or her blood sugar or cholesterol levels without first talking to a qualified medical doctor.

What else should I know about chromium supplements?

Short-term use of chromium supplements hasn't been associated with major side effects other than stomach upset. But there have been reports of anemia, cognitive problems, and other health disturbances in people who used high doses of chromium for extended periods. Little is known about the long-term effects of taking chromium supplements. It's possible that this metal could accumulate in the body, leading to serious health problems. One report suggested that the most widely used form, chromium picolinate, caused DNA damage in a test-tube analysis. Other lab studies have shown that related forms of chromium can damage DNA and cause cancer.

Chromium might interfere with medication intended to control blood-sugar levels.

Bottom line

Like many nonprescription weight-loss aids, chromium hasn't been adequately studied. There are safer ways to shed pounds than taking a supplement with a questionable record of efficacy and safety.

COENZYME Q$_{10}$

Also known as CoQ$_{10}$ (pronounced "ko-kyoo ten") and ubiquinone

What is it?

This vitamin-like substance is nearly ubiquitous in the human body, which explains coenzyme Q$_{10}$'s other name, ubiquinone. CoQ$_{10}$ is found in every human cell, where it is vital for the production of energy. CoQ$_{10}$ is also a powerful antioxidant. Minute amounts of CoQ$_{10}$ are found in many foods; rich sources include beef, soy oil, sardines, mackerel, and peanuts. CoQ$_{10}$ dietary supplements are usually sold as capsules.

Why do some people take CoQ$_{10}$ supplements?

CoQ$_{10}$ appears to be most commonly used by people who have, or want to prevent, heart disease. It has gained an especially strong reputation for the self-treatment of congestive heart failure. In this condition, weakened heart muscle struggles to pump enough blood to the lungs and muscles, causing fatigue and breathlessness.

CoQ$_{10}$ supplements are also touted as beneficial for many other conditions, including cancer, gum disease, male infertility, and neurological disorders. Some athletes believe it improves performance, too.

Do they work?

Despite the enthusiastic support for CoQ$_{10}$ voiced in several popular books, there is still no conclusive proof that this supplement treats or prevents congestive heart failure or any other form of cardiovascular disease. Some doctors have theorized that CoQ$_{10}$ might provide a weakened heart with an energy boost. But research findings so far have been inconsistent.

For example, a 1993 Italian study involving over six hundred heart failure patients suggests that taking CoQ$_{10}$ supplements might prevent the condition from worsening. On the other hand, doctors at the University of Maryland found that giving CoQ$_{10}$ supplements to heart failure patients didn't improve the amount of blood their hearts pumped, or how long they could exercise.

Some scientists believe that CoQ$_{10}$'s antioxidant punch might prevent artery damage that leads to heart disease in the first place. But no satisfactory studies have ever shown that taking these supplements prevents heart attacks. Likewise, there's not enough evidence to support the use of CoQ$_{10}$ for any other medical condition. However, trials conducted in the United States will test the hypothesis that CoQ$_{10}$ might benefit patients with two devastating neurological disorders, Parkinson's and Huntington's diseases, by restoring life to damaged cerebral cells.

Finally, does CoQ$_{10}$ improve athletic performance? It's an attractive theory, since CoQ$_{10}$ plays a key role in producing energy. But the studies are equivocal, at best, and several have found that the vitamin-like substance won't make you run any faster or longer.

What else should I know about CoQ_{10} supplements?

CoQ_{10} is thought to be safe in large doses, but the long-term effects of CoQ_{10} supplementation have not been studied. It is known that some users experience minor discomfort, such as an upset stomach.

Bottom line

There's currently not enough known about CoQ_{10} to recommend its use, particularly for the treatment of heart failure. If you frequently lack energy, schedule a checkup with your physician, soon.

CRANBERRY EXTRACT

Scientific name: *Vaccinium macrocarpon* and other species

What is it?

The humble, rather bitter-tasting cranberry plays a critical role in traditional American cuisine. After all, no Thanksgiving dinner is complete without cranberry sauce or relish. Although some species grow in the wild, most cranberries consumed in the United States come from commercial bogs, primarily in Wisconsin, Massachusetts, New Jersey, and the Pacific Northwest. Many of those berries are destined to be pressed and sold as cranberry juice, of course. The juice is sometimes used to flavor teas and is also dried and sold in capsule form as cranberry extract.

Why do some people take cranberry extract supplements?

To prevent and treat urinary tract infections, or UTIs. Generations of women have used cranberry juice as homemade medicine to avoid repeat episodes of this problem, which is caused by bacteria in the urethra, bladder, or kidneys. (Young and middle-aged females are fifty times more likely than males to develop UTIs, though the ratio evens out in later years.) Symptoms include a frequent need to urinate, often accompanied by a burning sensation and producing small amounts of cloudy, pungent urine. Cranberry extract supplements are marketed as a convenient way to get the benefits of cranberry juice, without all the calories.

Does it work?

There is a limited amount of evidence that the cranberry juice cure may be worth a try. In a 1994 experiment, Harvard researchers found that 15 percent of elderly women who drank nine ounces of the juice every day had evidence of a urinary infection, while 28 percent of women who drank a similar-tasting placebo beverage developed UTIs. The effect, however, was noted after one to two months of consuming the juice and it's worth noting that few of the women had symptoms of a urinary infection when the study began. Scientists once thought the acidity of cranberry juice killed bacteria, though it now appears as though some chemical in the fruit may make it difficult for the infectious microbes to adhere to the lining of the urinary tract.

But does that mean that pills containing cranberry extract have the same effect? Changing the composition of a substance—in this case, turning cranberry juice into a dried concentrate—may alter the way it behaves. One very small study suggests that cranberry extract supplements are at least worthy of more study. Researchers recruited a small group of women—just ten completed the study—each of whom had a history of UTIs. Taking daily cranberry supplements appeared to reduce the occurrence of infections, but a larger clinical trial would be needed to confirm their benefits.

What else should I know about cranberry extract supplements?

Most people can eat fresh cranberries and drink cranberry juice without experiencing any obvious side effects, though little is known about use of the pills. One place they might cause a little pain is your wallet. A month's supply of cranberry extract may cost as much as $20 or more, making it considerably more expensive than the juice.

Fever and back pain that accompany a burning sensation when urinating may be signs of a serious infection. UTIs can even be life threatening, especially in older women, requiring immediate attention and treatment with antibiotics.

Bottom line

A limited amount of research suggests that consuming cranberry for a prolonged period may decrease bacteria levels in the urine, which may in turn reduce the risk of a urinary tract infection. However, cranberry's therapeutic value needs further study. If you develop the symptoms of a UTI, see your physician.

CREATINE

Also known as creatine monohydrate

What is it?

Creatine is an amino acid that plays an important role in fueling muscle movement. Your body manufactures some of its own creatine, with the remainder coming from the diet. Several foods—particularly beef, dairy products, and fish—are good sources. However, people who use creatine supplements often take at least 20 grams per day. By some estimates, you would need to eat ten pounds of steak to get that much creatine. This supplement is usually sold as a powdered drink mix, though pills, liquids, and even creatine candy and chewing gum are available.

Why do some people take creatine supplements?

To build bigger muscles and gain physical strength. Creatine has been the most popular sports supplement in the United States since the mid-1990s. It became a topic of controversy when brawny baseball slugger Mark McGwire told reporters he used creatine (along with another supplement, androstenedione) in 1998, during his pursuit of Babe Ruth's single-season home run record.

Do they work?

The science isn't unanimous, but many studies suggest that creatine supplements help build bigger muscles. Since creatine can transfer energy to muscle, scientists theorize that loading up muscles with extra stores of the amino acid allows users to train longer and harder. For example, a 1997 study found that male weight lifters who consumed 25 grams of creatine per day for one week were able to do significantly more bench presses than counterparts who didn't take the supplement. Their strength appeared to increase faster, too.

Several other studies show that creatine can help build strength and boost muscle size. However, creatine's track record for actually improving athletic performance is uneven, at best. Studies of cyclists, swimmers, sprinters, and rowers have yielded inconsistent results—some showed improved times and speed, while in others creatine appeared to offer no benefit. Since creatine is involved in the production of anaerobic energy—the kind needed for short, intense bursts of activity—it may be of no use to long-distance runners and other athletes involved in longer, low-intensity activities, which use aerobic energy.

A few other caveats. Some research shows that creatine will not help about 20–30 percent of people who try it, possibly because their muscles are already "saturated" with the amino acid. Most studies of this supplement to date have involved young, well-trained men; less is known about whether women or the elderly can benefit from creatine. Finally, creatine is not like Popeye's spinach. Simply taking the supplement is a waste of time if you don't work out; without exercising your muscles will not magically grow larger.

What else should I know about creatine supplements?

Most studies of creatine have only lasted a few weeks; little is known about the safety of long-term use of this supplement. Some users have complained of dehydration and muscle tears, though it's not clear these problems were caused by creatine.

Creatine users can count on gaining a few pounds; there's some debate whether the added weight comes from new muscle, water retained in muscle cells, or both.

Bottom line

Studies suggest that creatine may help build muscle, but little is known about the safety of using this supplement.

DHEA

Scientific name: dehydroepiandrosterone

What is it?

DHEA is a hormone, which is a chemical compound that travels through the body from one tissue to another, causing some physiological change. Hormones regulate many aspects of human biology, including growth, metabolism, and reproduction. But while the adrenal gland produces large quantities of DHEA (along with a related compound, DHEA-S, or dehydroepiandrosterone sulfate), this hormone's role in human health isn't clear. However, DHEA is sometimes called the mother steroid, since it's a precursor, or building block, for two important hormones, testosterone and estradiol. Scientists also know that DHEA levels peak in early adulthood and decline with age in both men and women.

A typical diet provides negligible amounts of DHEA. Supplements are sold as capsules and tablets.

Why do some people take DHEA supplements?

DHEA has been touted as a fountain of youth or antiaging compound. Some people take these supplements in the belief that boosting levels will help trim expanding waistlines and rebuild lost muscle. Others use DHEA to sharpen their minds or ward off conditions associated with aging, such as heart disease and erectile dysfunction. DHEA has also been studied for the treatment of certain diseases, such as lupus erythematosus and HIV.

Do they work?

It's an appealing theory: Middle-agers and the elderly can rediscover the bloom and vigor of youth simply by restoring depleted DHEA. Unfortunately, matters of human biology are rarely that simple, and tinkering with hormone levels is no exception. For starters, overloading the body with DHEA, in the form of supplements, doesn't always produce elevated blood levels of the hormone. And even when it does, the benefits of boosted DHEA aren't clear.

Example: Some scientists have theorized that DHEA could act like anabolic steroids, producing growth in muscle tissue. But while an early study found that taking the supplements helped men drop fat and bulk up, subsequent research has failed to duplicate those findings. DHEA has only been shown to produce weight loss in animals, particularly lab rats. But that probably doesn't mean much to humans, since rats naturally produce very little DHEA.

Some studies suggest that men with cardiovascular disease have lower than expected amounts of circulating DHEA. But no one knows yet whether these low hormone levels are the cause or result of heart disease. A preliminary study of men with erectile dysfunction (ED) found that subjects who took DHEA showed great improvement in symptoms for the duration of the trial, which was six months. In the same study, men taking placebo pills showed initial improvement, but developed ED again after a few months. However, the authors concede that the potential benefits of DHEA need to be examined in a larger group of subjects.

DHEA's reputation as brain food comes from more animal studies, which suggest that the compound may improve certain aspects of memory and protect neuronal cells. But measurements of DHEA levels and cognitive performance have produced mixed results, with many finding no association between the hormone and brainpower. In fact, one recent study found that declining levels of DHEA in men had no effect on their ability to think and recall.

Before you get the idea that DHEA has no valid role in medicine, consider that research on the hormone is still in its infancy. And that it shows promise in several areas. Recent research suggests that DHEA may be a viable treatment for the immune system condition known as lupus erythematosus. There is also evidence that supplementation with DHEA may improve mood and sexual interest in women whose adrenal glands produce low levels of DHEA due to certain medical conditions or procedures. Of course, treatment of both of these serious conditions requires a medical doctor's supervision.

Some researchers have tried to determine whether DHEA has a role in treating or preventing cancer, but no conclusions can be drawn from studies performed so far. It's important to point out that manipulating hormone levels by any means in the human body carries the risk of serious side effects—and should not be done without a physician's guidance. For example, DHEA may raise levels of the so-called male hormone, testosterone—which could, in theory, increase the risk of prostate cancer. Similarly, any substance that raises levels of the hormone estrogen could increase the risk (again, in theory) of breast cancer.

What else should I know about DHEA supplements?

Reported side effects in studies of DHEA are uncommon, but it should nonetheless be regarded with caution. The safety of this hormone supplement hasn't been properly studied, and could have unhealthy consequences. For example, since the presence of DHEA may increase testosterone levels, women who use this supplement may grow facial hair. Their levels of HDL ("good") cholesterol could drop, too, which could increase the risk of heart disease.

Bottom line

Too little is known about DHEA to say whether it's safe and effective. However, it may alter hormone levels in men and women, which could lead to serious health hazards.

DONG QUAI

Scientific name: *Angelica sinensis*

What is it?

This plant grows on cold, damp mountain slopes in China, Japan, and Korea. The dried root has been a mainstay of traditional medicine in Asia for about two thousand years. As a dietary supplement, dong quai is usually sold in capsule form, but is also prepared as liquid extract, teas, and powders. The herb is also beginning to turn up in some less likely products, including cosmetics and linen spray.

Why do some people take dong quai supplements?

Dong quai is sometimes called women's ginseng, since herbalists recommend it for virtually any gynecological problem. It is said to ease menstrual cramps and PMS, while acting as an invigorating tonic during the menstrual period. Dong quai also allegedly reduces hot flashes and other symptoms in women who have reached menopause.

Do they work?

Dong quai has been widely used in the United States for only a few years, so it's not surprising that there has been little research on the herb conducted here. However, a 1997 study attempted to determine whether dong quai offers any benefits to women who are bothered by hot flashes and other postmenopausal symptoms. A group of seventy-one women with these complaints were divided into two groups. One received 4.5 grams of dong quai root daily for six months; the other was given a look-alike pill that contained no herbs. In the end, the researchers determined that dong quai was no better than a placebo for relieving menopausal symptoms.

The authors of the study anticipated one possible criticism of their work: A traditional Chinese healer would probably recommend dong quai in combination with some other herb or herbs. However, dong quai is often sold alone, not blended with other herbs, in the United States.

Although not conclusive, this study offers reason to doubt whether dong quai preparations are worth the money—and the potential risk—unless further research proves them to be safe and effective (see next section).

Too little is known about dong quai for the treatment of cramps and other symptoms related to menstruation to recommend it for that purpose. And there's no reason to think that rubbing on body lotions containing dong quai, or spritzing the herb on your bed sheets, will confer any health benefits.

What else should I know about dong quai supplements?

No major side effects were reported in the study mentioned earlier, though this herb may have a mild laxative effect on some users. Dong quai contains several compounds that may interfere with prescription blood thinners, which could lead to internal bleeding.

Although the evidence is not clear, some literature suggests that dong quai has some of the same properties as the female hormone estrogen. This offers another reason to view this herb with caution, since altering estrogen levels may increase the risk of some cancers (such as uterine cancer), which is why any kind of hormone therapy must be administered by a physician. Pregnant women should beware of herbs that contain hormones, since they could cause spontaneous abortion. (See the separate entry for soy, p. 178, to read more about plant estrogens and their health benefits and risks.)

Some constituents of dong quai can also make skin extrasensitive to sunlight, causing severe rashes, and may even be carcinogenic.

Bottom line

There is no clear evidence that dong quai does what its promoters claim. Furthermore, it may contain potentially harmful substances. Talk to your physician about other ways to control postmenopausal symptoms.

ECHINACEA

Scientific names: *Echinacea angustifolia, E. pallida,* and *E. purpurea*
Pronounced "ek-ih-NAY-shuh"

What is it?

This plant, native to the American Midwest, was first used by the Plains Indians to heal wounds and treat infections. Echinacea eventually became a popular pharmaceutical product in the United States, though it fell out of favor when antibiotics were introduced in the 1930s. However, about a generation ago interest in this perennial's therapeutic value stirred anew. Today, doctors write about 2.5 million prescriptions each year for echinacea in Germany, where the herb is used like a drug. Echinacea is available over-the-counter in the United States, and in recent years has become one of the top-selling medicinal herbs.

Three different species of echinacea are used medicinally, though *Echinacea purpurea* is the most widely studied and sold. The roots, stems, and pinkish-purple flowers may be processed for commercial herbal supplements, which come in many forms, including capsules, liquid drops, juice, and teas. Echinacea is frequently blended with other medicinal herbs.

Why do some people take echinacea supplements?

To prevent the onset of an upper respiratory infection, which you know better as the common cold. Echinacea is also used as a cold therapy, taken to make the symptoms more bearable and disappear speedily if you do catch a case of the sniffles. Some people take echinacea all year round in the belief that it helps build a healthy immune system.

Do they work?

A handful of studies have suggested that echinacea may help limit your chance of catching a cold, but don't toss out your handkerchief just yet. Much of the research that helped build this herb's reputation as a cold fighter doesn't meet the standards used in the United States to determine if a drug is safe and effective. Meanwhile, when echinacea has been tested under strict scientific standards, doubts have arisen about how well it prevents colds and relieves their symptoms. One study found it to be no more effective than sugar pills. In another, people who took echinacea were less likely to catch a cold—but not by much. According to one estimate, this herb may only reduce the risk for upper respiratory infections by 10–20 percent.

Some laboratory studies have shown that echinacea may stimulate the immune system. But how, or whether, the herb should be used for that purpose isn't known.

What else should I know about echinacea supplements?

People have been taking this herb in Europe and the United States for years, with no serious side effects reported. Still, long-term studies of echinacea haven't been conducted, and health officials in Germany discourage its use for longer than eight weeks. Echinacea may interfere with immunosuppressive drugs, such as cyclosporine and any of the corticosteroids.

Although *Echinacea purpurea* is the most extensively studied species of echinacea, it's not always possible to determine which variety was used to produce a given brand, since manufacturers aren't required to say so on labels.

To reduce the odds that you'll catch a cold, get plenty of rest and wash your hands frequently. And go ahead and get rid of that handkerchief; instead of carrying around a piece of germ-laden linen, blow your nose with disposable tissues instead.

Bottom line

Although some studies suggest that taking echinacea may shorten the duration of cold symptoms, more research is needed to determine whether this herb offers safe, effective therapy. And while it may have some effect on the immune system, it's not clear what that is, or whether that effect is even good for human health.

ENZYME FORMULAS

Sometimes called digestive or proteolytic enzymes; also identified as bromelain, papain, and other names

What are they?

Enzymes are catalysts. In the human body, these specialized proteins initiate and speed up chemical reactions that keep your internal machinery running. One of the many important functions of enzymes is to help digest food by breaking down carbohydrates, fat, and protein into smaller components that can be absorbed into the bloodstream. Your body manufactures enzymes, and they're found in some foods, too. Enzyme supplements—some derived from animal organs, others from certain fruits—are sold as tablets, capsules, and powdered beverages.

Why do some people take enzyme supplements?

Proponents of enzyme therapy claim that high doses of these proteins can improve human health in myriad ways, but the supplements are most commonly marketed as digestive aids. Some boosters go even farther, claiming that enzyme supplements can reduce the risk of heart attacks and strokes, relieve back pain and arthritis, diminish swelling, fight cancer and HIV/AIDS, and even sharpen your wits.

Do they work?

Some common medical conditions are associated with missing or low levels of certain digestive enzymes, including lactose intolerance, cystic fibrosis, and pancreatitis. Supplementary enzymes are often prescribed to patients with the symptoms of these conditions; a simple example would be over-the-counter lactase pills, which replace the enzyme missing in people with lactose intolerance, allowing them to consume dairy products.

However, many claims made by companies that sell enzyme supplements lack evidence to back them up. One frequent refrain argues that modern food-processing techniques rob foods of natural enzymes. As one theory goes, that leaves some people with inadequate levels of enzymes in their intestines to fully break down food. The resulting undigested gunk lingering in the GI tract is said to cause pain, bloating, and other symptoms of dyspepsia, or indigestion. But there's no scientific proof to support this theory.

Furthermore, common claims that undigested food particles cause allergies that are responsible for various illnesses are, to say the least, hard to swallow. The same is true for the argument that certain enzymes will break down fat in the blood, and thus trim your waistline and protect you from heart disease. The fact is, digestive enzymes are only active in the bowel; they break down before being absorbed into the bloodstream, making it inconceivable that they would have any affect on cholesterol or other lipids in the blood.

What else should I know about enzyme supplements?

Lacking long-term studies, no one can say whether taking enzyme supplements on a regular basis is safe. If you suffer from frequent indigestion, talk to your physician.

Bottom line

Digestive enzymes prescribed by physicians are useful in the treatment of specific medical conditions. However, claims made about enzyme supplements sold in health food stores and on the Internet lack proof; some don't even make physiological sense.

EPHEDRA

Scientific names: *Ephedra sinica, E. equisetina*, and *E. intermedia*
Also known as ma huang

What is it?

Many species of ephedra grow all over the world, but those commonly found in herbal products are native to India, Pakistan, and China. The dried stems and roots of this shrub have been used in traditional Chinese medicine for over five thousand years. Ephedra contains many different alkaloids, or active ingredients, including the drugs ephedrine and pseudoephedrine. The latter is a familiar ingredient in cold and allergy remedies, though the vast majority of these products sold in the United States contain a man-made version of pseudoephedrine. Likewise, synthetic ephedrine is a prescription medicine for the treatment of asthma.

As a dietary supplement, ephedra is sold in tablet, capsule, powder, and liquid forms, often blended with other herbs.

Why do some people take ephedra supplements?

Ephedra is used primarily in this country as a weight-loss aid and energy booster. By one estimate, Americans take 3 billion servings of ephedra each year. It's also used in traditional Chinese medicine for nasal decongestion and asthma; the often-quoted Commission E, Germany's authority on the use of herbal medicine, has approved the use of ephedra to treat coughs and bronchitis.

Do they work?

A few studies have shown that taking the alkaloid ephedrine while dieting may cause a modest weight loss, especially if it's consumed with caffeine. However, there are several caveats about these studies. More important, anyone who considers using ephedra supplements must recognize that these products carry serious health risks.

First, the caveats. Most research on the weight-reducing effects of ephedrine has involved small groups of subjects who were given a synthetic version of the alkaloid. Meanwhile, there has been very little research on the herb ephedra as a diet aid. In one six-month trial, published in 2001, people who took a preparation of ephedra and the herb guarana (a source of caffeine) lost six pounds more than dieters who weren't given the herbs. However, nearly a quarter of the patients who took ephedra supplements dropped out of the study because of unpleasant side-effects; more on that later.

No one is sure why the alkaloid ephedrine causes weight loss, though it may suppress appetite or speed up metabolism, effects that appear to be

enhanced by caffeine. What's more, weight lost through the use of a stimulant—whether it's an over-the-counter diet drug or an herb such as
ephedra—is rarely permanent; the pounds often return within a few weeks
or months.

As mentioned, scientists have long known that ephedra can cause
unpleasant side effects. What's more, the Food and Drug Administration
has compiled dozens of reports of fatal heart attacks, strokes, and deaths
by other causes associated with use of this herb. Still, defenders of
ephedra within the dietary supplements industry argue that it's safe
when used in the proper dosages by people who don't have heart disease
or other certain medical conditions.

However, the FDA commissioned an independent analysis of
"adverse events" in people who took ephedra that the agency received
between 1997 and 1999. Not only did the authors of the report attrib-
ute ten deaths and thirteen cases of permanent disability to the use of
products that contain ephedra, but they also suggested that even modest
intake of ephedra can be risky, for anyone. The authors turned up evidence that at least nine people who were healthy and using relatively low
doses of ephedra alkaloids (which they defined as 12–36 milligrams of
ephedra alkaloids per day) suffered serious medical problems. Furthermore, the authors noted that eleven heart attacks and strokes occurred
in people with no previously reported health conditions.

Regardless of Commission E's stance, ephedra shouldn't be used as a
nasal decongestant or to treat any kind of bronchial problem. It hasn't
been well studied for these purposes, while there are many over-the-
counter and prescription cold remedies and allergy medications available
that have been exhaustively tested. (However, it's still a good idea to discuss the use of nasal decongestants with your physician, since some of
these drugs contain ingredients that may affect certain medical conditions; for example, products that contain pseudoephedrine may be inappropriate for some people with high blood pressure.)

What else should I know about ephedra supplements?

Ephedra is a potent stimulant that acts like adrenaline in the body,
revving up the heart and brain. (It's often found in "herbal Ecstasy"
preparations, which are so-called natural alternatives to the street drug

Ecstasy.) Some common side effects reported by people who use ephedra include heart palpitations, nervousness, irritability, and insomnia. These effects could be heightened in people who take prescription antidepressants known as MAO inhibitors. Diabetics who take medication to control blood sugar shouldn't use ephedra.

As with many dietary supplements, the amount of active ingredient listed on the label of an ephedra bottle may not match the actual content of the pills or powder inside. Researchers at the University of Arkansas measured the ephedrine levels in twenty different commercially available supplements. They found that half the products contained more or less ephedrine than claimed on the labels, with discrepancies reaching up to 20 percent.

Bottom line

This herb contains compounds that are similar to amphetamine drugs, which are strong cardiovascular and central-nervous-system stimulants. Ephedra supplements have the potential to cause life-threatening health risks. They should not be used for any purpose.

ESSENTIAL FATTY ACIDS

Often abbreviated as EFA

What are they?

Essential fatty acids, or EFAs, are sometimes referred to as "good" fats. Unlike saturated fat and trans fatty acids, which appear to raise the risk of heart disease and other conditions, essential fatty acids are necessary for human health. They not only provide the body with energy, but also perform several other important jobs. One is to serve as components for prostaglandins, hormonelike substances that play a number of critical roles in the body.

Humans can't synthesize these fatty acids, which makes them an "essential" part of a healthy diet. Two of the main sources are vegetable oils and seafood. Deficiency of essential fatty acids has been associated with learning disabilities, vision problems, excessive thirst, stunted growth, skin and liver disorders, and infertility.

EFA formula supplements are usually sold as capsules or liquid and may include two or more of a long list of oils and other sources of fat, which may include (but is not limited to):

alpha-linolenic acid, or ALA
black currant seed oil
borage seed oil
bran oil
conjugated linoleic acid, or CLA
docosahexaenoic acid, or DHA
evening primrose oil
fish oil
flaxseed oil
gamma-linolenic acid, or GLA
medium-chain triglycerides
oleic acid
pumpkin seed oil
rice germ oil
rosemary oil
safflower oil
sesame oil
sunflower oil
wheat germ oil

Why do some people take essential fatty acid supplements?

Supplement sellers suggest through marketing that EFA supplements add life to skin and hair, relieve joint pain, lower levels of cholesterol and other blood fats, reduce blood pressure, and help the cardiovascular system in other ways.

Do they work?

Proponents claim that many people—up to 80 percent of Americans, according to *The Encyclopedia of Natural Medicine*—suffer from a deficiency of EFAs. Adding EFAs to the diet, they say, may prevent or treat many common diseases and conditions, including arthritis, eczema, and heart disease. But the suggestion that such a large portion of the population doesn't consume adequate amounts of EFAs is highly controversial and isn't backed by solid scientific evidence. Diagnosed cases of EFA deficiency can be treated with supplements, but this condition is rare.

Furthermore, it's difficult to make general statements about EFAs as a category, since supplement companies use so many different oil extracts to create their own individual formulas. However, some individual EFAs have been studied and may one day prove to have some therapeutic use. See separate entries for evening primrose oil (page 81), fish oil (page 89), and flaxseed (page 92).

What else should I know about essential fatty acid supplements?

Fat supplies twice as many calories per gram as protein and carbohydrates. A single EFA capsule may contain only a modest amount of fat, but if you take several per day, as many manufacturers recommend, the calories could begin to add up.

Although the therapeutic value of these supplements hasn't been proven, there are good reasons to add foods rich in EFAs to your diet. EFAs are polyunsaturated fats, which do not increase the risk of heart disease. Foods that are high in polyunsaturated fats, such as fish, can replace red meat and other foods that are high in artery-clogging saturated fats. (However, if you see the word *hydrogenated* on a food label, beware; that means it contains polyunsaturated fats that have been processed in a way that makes them act more like unhealthy saturated fats.) Many public health authorities recommend eating a diet that includes less than 30 percent of total calories as fat, with no more than 7–10 percent in the form of saturated fat. Ask your physician for specific recommendations about your dietary needs.

Bottom line

Replacing saturated fat in your diet with polyunsaturated fats may reduce the risk of heart disease. But there are no proven benefits to consuming EFA supplements.

EVENING PRIMROSE OIL

Scientific name: *Oenothera biennis*
Sometimes abbreviated as EPO

What is it?

The evening primrose is a plant with large yellow flowers that's found throughout North America, particularly in the East. (Any botanist can tell you, however, that it's not a true primrose, which belongs to another plant family.) The seeds of evening primrose produce an oil that contains several essential fatty acids, including one called gamma-linolenic acid, or GLA. Evening primrose oil supplements are sold as capsules and liquid extract.

Why do some people take evening primrose oil supplements?

Herbalists recommend this oil for the treatment of many conditions, especially arthritis, eczema and other skin problems, and symptoms of PMS (premenstrual syndrome).

Do they work?

Although there are no conclusive answers, some evidence suggests that evening primrose oil might help relieve the symptoms of a few conditions that involve inflammation. According to one theory, raising the levels of GLA in the body leads to the production of a certain type of prostaglandin that stops inflammation. In a few small studies, some people with rheumatoid arthritis who took supplements containing GLA had less joint pain, swelling, and stiffness than people who were given dummy pills. Evening primrose oil and other sources of GLA do not appear to be strong enough medicine to replace non-steroidal anti-inflammatory drugs (NSAIDs), which are standard therapy for rheumatoid arthritis. However, a few people in these studies were able to cut back on the amount of NSAIDs they used.

Evening primrose oil has been studied for treatment of a few skin conditions, including atopic dermatitis, a type of rash caused by inflammation. However, many dermatologists remain skeptical about its value. If you're bothered by PMS, evening primrose oil may not be the answer to your problems. Only a few small studies have examined whether the oil offers any benefit to women with PMS, and the overall results aren't very encouraging. However, it may relieve a specific symptom, mastalgia, or painful breasts, which affects some women during menstruation, though closer study is needed to determine whether evening primrose oil is safe and effective for this purpose.

What else should I know about evening primrose oil supplements?

Not much is known about the safety of consuming evening primrose oil. While it appears to be relatively nontoxic, there have been reports of seizures in some users. (People who use anticonvulsive drugs should avoid evening primrose oil.) Furthermore, there is reason to suspect that this oil could be toxic in other ways. For example, if evening primrose does relieve breast pain, that suggests that it could contain hormones or hormonelike substances—which could, theoretically, have detrimental effects. For example, excess estrogen may increase the risk of breast or uterine cancer.

Some reported side effects include nausea, headache, and soft stools. All fatty acids are concentrated sources of calories. Pop too many pills containing evening primrose oil, or any other oil, and you may feel the effects in your waistline, too.

See the separate entry for essential fatty acids (page 78).

Bottom line

Evening primrose oil may help relieve some painful conditions associated with inflammation, but can't be recommended, due to the lack of data on its safety and effectiveness.

EYEBRIGHT

Scientific name: *Euphrasia officinalis*

What is it?

There are several plants called eyebright, but *Euphrasia officinalis* is the variety commonly recommended by herbalists. It grows primarily in Europe and has been used as medicine since at least the Middle Ages. Eyebright is sold in several forms, including pills and powders (sometimes blended with other dietary supplements, including bilberry and lutein—see separate entries), teas, and eye lotions.

Why do some people take eyebright supplements?

To improve vision and treat just about any eye affliction, from simple irritation to conjunctivitis. Some herbalists recommend it for sinus problems, too.

Do they work?

To some observers' eyes, flower petals on the eyebright plant can appear "bloodshot," since they sometimes produce red spots and streaks. For centuries, and even today, that botanical quirk alone has inspired the use of this herb to improve sight and treat eye ailments. In other words, there's not a shred of scientific evidence in Western medical literature to recommend the use of eyebright, in any form or for any purpose. In fact, applying an eyewash created at home could carry significant dangers (see next section).

What else should I know about eyebright supplements?

There's no way of knowing whether this herb is safe or not. Homemade eyewashes, using eyebright or any other herb, are generally a bad idea, since they may contain irritants that could damage your eyes.

Bottom line

If you have vision problems, don't self-treat them with this unproven herb—or any herb, for that matter. See a physician instead.

FEVERFEW

Scientific name: *Tanacetum parthenium*

What is it?

Feverfew is a short, daisylike plant with yellow flowers that grows in parts of North America, Europe, and Australia. The feathery leaves of the feverfew are used as medicine. Its name is adapted from a Latin word that means "fever reducer." Feverfew supplements are usually sold as capsules or tablets, though drops are available, too.

Why do some people take feverfew supplements?

Despite its name, feverfew is thought of most often today as an herb for preventing migraine headaches. More than 3 million women and 1 million men in the United States suffer at least one migraine attack per month. In Canada, feverfew is sold as an approved over-the-counter drug for treating these severe headaches, which are often accompanied by other symptoms, such as nausea.

Some herbalists also recommend feverfew for the relief of pain associated with rheumatoid arthritis.

Do they work?

Lab studies suggest that feverfew may reduce inflammation and bring about other chemical changes that would help control headaches. Some scientific interest in this herb has focused on its content of a substance called parthenolide. But, despite winning approval by Canadian authorities, the evidence for feverfew's value for treating migraines is rather modest. According to one of the few controlled trials to study migraine sufferers who took feverfew, the herb reduced the frequency of attacks by 24 percent, but did nothing to minimize the severity of attacks. There have been a few other studies of feverfew and migraineurs, but they've either involved small groups of subjects or had serious design flaws. In short, further research, involving larger groups of subjects, is needed to draw firm conclusions about feverfew.

Feverfew's ability to control pain in people with rheumatoid arthritis has not been extensively studied, but the authors of one trial determined that a daily dose of up to 86 milligrams of feverfew did nothing to relieve stiffness and pain or improve grip strength.

What else should I know about feverfew supplements?

Nothing is known about the safety of using feverfew for a long period, since the duration of most studies on the herb has been brief. If you're allergic to ragweed or other members of the *Compositae* family, you may be allergic to feverfew, too. Some people who try feverfew develop mouth sores and/or gastrointestinal problems. Quitting this herb may cause "rebound" headaches, as well as nervousness, insomnia, and other symptoms. Some studies suggest that feverfew may interact with drugs used to prevent blood clotting. If your doctor has instructed you to take iron supplements, beware that feverfew may make them harder for your body to absorb.

Bottom line

Feverfew has not been proven to be an effective and safe preventive or treatment for migraine headache. If you're plagued by this often-debilitating problem, talk to a physician about lifestyle changes and new medications that may help.

FIBER SUPPLEMENTS

What are they?

All plant foods—fruits, vegetables, seeds, and grains—contain material that can't be broken down by enzymes in the human digestive system. Fiber, or "roughage," as your mother may have called it, passes through the body without being absorbed. But while it's not technically a nutrient, fiber plays several vital roles in human nutrition nonetheless. For example, it sops up water and moves swiftly through the intestine, which aids digestion. Fiber also plays a role in controlling cholesterol levels.

Although all plants contain fiber (which gives them shape and structure), there are a few particularly dense sources. Wheat and oat bran are perhaps the best-known examples, but one of the most widely used plants in dietary supplements is the lesser-known psyllium, which is prized for its seed husks. You may be familiar with the phrases "soluble fiber" and "insoluble fiber." As its name suggests, soluble fiber dissolves better in water, meaning that it soaks up more water in the digestive tract. Some scientists believe that soluble fiber provides greater health benefits, though that theory remains controversial.

Fiber supplements are sold in many forms, including powdered beverages, granules (which are placed on the tongue and washed down with water), wafers, and chewable tablets.

Why do some people take fiber supplements?

In polite company, it's called keeping regular—that is, to prevent and treat constipation. People suffering from other gastrointestinal problems, such as diverticulosis and irritable bowel syndrome, may also use fiber supplements. So-called colon cleanser products and some weight-loss aids often contain a source of fiber as the main ingredient. Fiber supplements are also used to lower the risk of more serious conditions, including heart disease, colon cancer, and diabetes.

Do they work?

Although the long-standing theory that fiber prevents colon cancer has been questioned in recent years, this quasi-nutrient has several important health benefits nonetheless. However, there is no question that a balanced diet—which includes plentiful servings of fruit, vegetables, and whole grains—is the ideal source of fiber. Unlike supplements, high-fiber foods are also packed with important vitamins, minerals, and micronutrients—and they taste better, too.

Still, fiber supplements can be useful in treating some conditions. For example, physicians may recommend adding psyllium to your diet to relieve occasional bouts with constipation. Psyllium's ability to soften and add bulk to the stool, which eases passage through the intestine, is well established. (Chronic constipation, meanwhile, may require prescription drugs that act on the bowel in other ways.) Fiber supplements are also sometimes used successfully in the management of diverticulosis (bulges in the intestine that may cause cramps and diarrhea) and irritable bowel syndrome (which causes abdominal pain and various gastrointestinal disturbances).

Avoid products sold in health food stores and on the Internet that promise to cleanse your colon. You don't need them and high doses of strong herbal laxatives are potentially dangerous (see next section).

Several studies have also shown that consuming fiber (from various sources, including psyllium) produces modest reductions in cholesterol, possibly by decreasing the amount of fats absorbed in the intestine. Some doctors suggest that their patients at risk for cardiovascular disease add small amounts of fiber from dietary supplements to their diets. However, the American Heart Association recommends consuming 25–30 grams of fiber each day—not from supplements, but food, which offers other healthful nutrients. Before taking fiber supplements to cut your risk for a heart attack, check if it's okay with your physician (especially if you're a diabetic, since some studies have suggested that adding fiber to the diet may change your insulin requirement).

Although doctors are studying the role of high-fiber diets in controlling obesity, dietary supplements containing fiber (often mixed with herbs) that are marketed as weight-loss aids have no proven value.

What else should I know about fiber supplements?

Abuse of any type of laxative can cause dehydration and the depletion of important minerals known as electrolytes, which could lead to heart trouble. It's especially important to discuss the use of laxatives with a physician if you're taking medication that regulates heart rhythm.

Don't self-treat chronic constipation; see a doctor instead. You may simply need to boost your fiber intake, but persistent bowel problems could signal the onset of a serious condition, such as an intestinal obstruction, ulcerative colitis, or appendicitis. In some cases, laxatives may only make things worse.

Going a day or two without a bowel movement on occasion isn't usually cause for alarm. However, if dealing with gastrointestinal discomfort has become part of your daily routine, talk to your physician.

Bottom line

Consuming fiber—especially from food—may reduce the risk of heart disease and have other health benefits. Eating a diet filled with fruits, vegetables, and whole-grain foods is a good start. To be sure you get the recommended 25–30 grams a day, see the box for tips on fibering up.

The American Heart Association and other health organizations recommend consuming at least 25 grams of fiber per day; most of us get about half that much. Eating more fruit and vegetables is an excellent start. You can also dramatically increase your fiber intake by making a few simple changes to your diet.

	Instead of ...	... choose	... and you'll gain this much fiber
Breakfast	I cup of corn flakes	I cup of oat bran	4.5 grams
Lunch	A sandwich made with two slices of white bread	A sandwich made with two slices of whole-wheat bread	3 grams
Snack	I chocolate bar	I apple	3 grams
Dinner	I cup white rice	I cup brown rice	2.5 grams
		Total increase in fiber intake	13 grams

All fiber values courtesy of *Bowes and Church's Food Values of Portions Commonly Used* (Lippincott, 1998)

FISH OIL

What is it?

If you're old enough, you may recall a time when mothers dosed virtually any malady with a spoonful or two of cod-liver oil. Children the world over should be glad that practice fell out of favor, yet the idea that fish oil contains medicine has enjoyed a renaissance in the last generation.

Fish oil contains omega-3 fatty acids, which belong to a larger category called the essential fatty acids. Your body, particularly the brain, needs essential fatty acids to function properly. But humans can't produce these vital fats on our own, so we have to get them from food. Dietary supplements containing oil pressed from cooked fish are sold as capsules. And, yes, you can even buy cod-liver oil gel-caps.

Why do some people take fish oil supplements?

Concern about the risk of heart disease is undoubtedly the leading reason Americans use fish oil supplements. However, recent scientific developments have spurred interest in using fish oil to treat other conditions, including rheumatoid arthritis and certain mental health problems.

Do they work?

In the 1970s, scientists noticed that the Eskimos of Greenland rarely develop heart disease. The typical Eskimo diet, which is very high in fat, made this finding all the more surprising. However, very little of the fat consumed by these hardy Greenlanders is the saturated kind that comes from beef and pork, which is associated with clogged arteries. Instead, Eskimos subsist largely on fish and seal meat, whose bodies are protected from icy waters by layers of polyunsaturated fat.

A theory quickly emerged: The specific type of polyunsaturated fat in fish, omega-3 fatty acids, may actually protect the heart. No one was sure how or why, but some researchers believed that omega-3's slowed production of cholesterol in the liver. Later studies have supported the idea that eating fish reduces the risk of a heart attack, although seafood is certainly no panacea. Some research suggests that there's probably little cardiovascular benefit to eating fish more than once or twice a week, and that only fatty fish (such as albacore tuna, bluefish, rainbow trout, and salmon) pack enough omega-3 fatty acids to do much good.

But does that mean fish oil capsules prevent heart disease? The question is still being studied, but evidence is emerging to suggest that they may. If that's true, it doesn't seem to be because fish oil lowers cholesterol. Instead, fish oil may have other benefits for the cardiovascular system. Some researchers believe that it stabilizes heart rhythm; according to one study, frequent fish eaters are half as likely to be victims of sudden cardiac death, which occurs when the heart begins beating erratically. Fish oil may also prevent blood clots, as well as reduce levels of blood fats known as triglycerides that are associated with an increased risk for heart disease—by as much as 30 percent, according to some studies. However, more research is needed to confirm these benefits.

For people who have already had heart attacks, the benefits of taking fish oil supplements to prevent arteries from reclogging is less clear. Some studies have shown that they might protect the heart, while others have found little or no benefit. However, a 1999 trial that included over eleven thousand people who had already had heart attacks found a lower risk of death, second heart attacks, and strokes among those who took fish oil capsules.

After prevention of heart disease, the most commonly studied therapeutic use of fish oil is probably the treatment of rheumatoid arthritis (RA). This painful joint disorder occurs when the body's immune system attacks its own tissue (unlike the more common osteoarthritis, which is caused by wear and tear on the joints). Some scientists theorize that omega-3 fatty acids stifle the production of prostaglandins, which cause inflammation. There have been a few small but promising studies in which patients with RA who took fish oil capsules along with their usual drug regimen had less joint stiffness and swelling; in some instances, patients felt good enough to decrease their drug dosage. However, it often took several months for patients to experience any benefits from fish oil supplements, and they usually took far larger doses than most manufacturers recommend. Furthermore, fish oil capsules haven't been compared head-to-head with state-of-the-art drugs now available for treating arthritis.

Some preliminary research hints that fish oil may be useful in the treatment of bipolar disorder and other psychiatric conditions, possibly by mimicking the activity of lithium and other psychoactive drugs. However, this area of study is still in its infancy. Likewise, a few studies suggest that people who eat lots of fish have a low risk for certain cancers, but whether they gain protection from seafood or some other influence is unknown.

Studies suggest that eating fish several times per week can lower the risk of cardiovascular disease. All varieties of seafood contain omega-3 fatty acids, but each of the following species is packed with at least 1 gram per serving (3.5 ounces) of this "good" fat.

Anchovies
Bluefish
Lake trout
Mackerel
Mullet
Sablefish
Salmon (Atlantic and Pacific)
Sardines

Note: The U.S. Food and Drug Administration has advised women who are pregnant or may become pregnant, nursing mothers, and young children not to eat certain species of fish that may contain high levels of mercury. These species are shark, swordfish, king mackerel, and tilefish. The FDA suggests that these groups of women and children should limit their fish intake to 12 ounces of cooked fish per week (a typical serving size is three to six ounces). Mercury may cause damage in developing brains that leads to learning disabilities.

The Environmental Protection Agency, meanwhile, warns that women who are pregnant or may become pregnant, nursing mothers, and young children should avoid fish caught in freshwater, which also may be contaminated with high levels of mercury. Be sure to talk to your physician about the proper role of fish in your family's diet.

What else should I know about fish oil supplements?

Taking high doses can give your breath a fishy odor. Some users develop loose stools and nausea, too. Oil is fat, which is a highly concentrated source of calories. If you currently take any type of blood-thinning medication, don't use fish oil capsules without your physician's consent.

Bottom line

Given the mounting evidence that they may prevent and treat heart disease and a few other conditions, fish oil capsules deserve further investigation of their therapeutic value and safety. However, it's not clear at present whether these supplements offer any advantages over a diet that includes frequent servings of fish.

FLAXSEED

Scientific name: *Linum usitatissimum*

What is it?

The versatile flax plant is grown in North America, Argentina, Russia, and Ukraine. Flax fibers are spun into linen cloth and its seeds are pressed to produce linseed oil, which is used in paints and varnishes. Leftover flaxseeds are crushed and ground to make livestock feed. As interest grows in flax's potential health benefits, many cooks today use the nutty tasting seeds (whole or ground into flour) and oil in a variety of recipes. Some commercial products, such as breads and breakfast cereals, are prepared with flaxseed, too. As a dietary supplement, flaxseed oil is sold by the bottle and in capsules. You can also pick up a bag of milled seeds at most health food stores.

Why do some people take flaxseed supplements?

Flaxseed currently enjoys a reputation as a super health food. Consumers take the supplement in hopes of reducing the risk of both heart disease and cancer. Some sources claim that flaxseed oil can relieve the symptoms of immune disorders, such as lupus, arthritis, and some allergies.

Do they work?

Many scientists are intrigued by the health-promoting potential of flaxseed, though more study is needed to understand this plant's role in fighting disease. For example, researchers have shown that flaxseed slows the spread of cancer cells in laboratory studies. If flaxseed turns out to have health-promoting benefits in humans, it could be due to chemicals called lignans, which may act as antioxidants and phytoestrogens (which are substances that mimic the hormone estrogen). But while no one can say whether flaxseed prevents cancer in humans, trials are under way. A team at the University of Toronto is studying whether a daily dose of flaxseed (baked into a muffin) slows the growth of tumors in women diagnosed with breast cancer.

A few studies involving humans have already looked at flaxseed as a defense against heart disease. In one, twenty-nine people with high cholesterol ate a daily muffin baked with flaxseed that had much of its oil removed. After three weeks, the subjects' blood was tested. Most had experienced slight decreases in total and LDL ("bad") cholesterol. Flaxseed is a rich source of omega-3 fatty acids, which are the kind some scientists believe make fish oil good for the heart. However, the cardiovascular benefits of flaxseed oil—which, obviously, has no fiber—haven't been well studied in clinical trials.

Dietary supplements containing omega-3 fatty acids, in the form of fish oil, have also been used to treat conditions caused by inflammation, particularly rheumatoid arthritis. Unfortunately, there has been relatively little research on flaxseed for the treatment of inflammatory disorders. One small study involving twenty-two patients found that flaxseed oil taken for three months offered no pain relief.

Like any other high-fiber food, a little flaxseed added to your diet may help clear up a case of constipation.

What else should I know about flax oil supplements?

No major side effects have been reported with consuming modest amounts of flaxseed. Still, it may affect the way medications are absorbed, so if you use these supplements, be sure your physician knows. Furthermore, according to some sources flaxseed contains compounds called cyanogenic glycosides, which could be poisonous. However, there do not appear to be any humans who developed toxic reactions to flaxseed.

Flaxseed has a laxative effect, which could be harmful in people who have bowel obstructions. Oil is liquid fat, and fat is a rich source of calories. Some companies recommend taking as many as ten flaxseed pills per day—which would add 600 calories to your weekly diet.

Bottom line

A high-fiber diet may decrease the risk of cancer and cardiovascular disease, but the value of flaxseed supplements and other alternative fiber sources is unclear. If you're considering this or any other supplement to treat constipation, see a physician first. Chronic bowel problems may be a sign of a more serious condition.

FOLIC ACID

Also known as folacin, folate, and vitamin B_9

What is it?

Folic acid is one of the B vitamins (see page 190). It plays an important role in growth and reproduction. Folic acid has several other functions; among the better known is its ability to remove a naturally occurring amino acid called homocysteine from the blood.

The word *folic* derives from the same Latin word as "foliage." Not surprisingly, leafy greens such as spinach and cabbage are among the best sources of the vitamin. Others include asparagus, broccoli, whole-grain breads and cereals, beans, oranges, peanuts, and organ meats. Furthermore, all grain products sold in the United States are enriched with folic acid. Most multivitamins contain 400 micrograms of folic acid, which is the recommended daily intake for adults (though requirements differ for women who are pregnant or lactating). Folic acid supplements are available, too.

Why do some people take folic acid supplements?

Pregnant women are often instructed to take folic acid supplements to reduce the fetus's risk for neural tube defects, such as spina bifida and other congenital diseases affecting the skull and spine. Some experts (notably physician Kilmer McCully, author of *The Heart Revolution*) have also begun recommending folic acid supplements to patients with very high blood levels of homocysteine.

Do they work?

Two large studies show that women who take folic acid supplements before and during pregnancy dramatically decrease the risk of giving birth to babies with neural tube defects. The Centers for Disease Control and Prevention recommends that women who may become pregnant consume 400 micrograms of folic acid a day. The CDC suggests eating plenty of foods that are rich in the vitamin, but taking a supplement if necessary. The safest bet: If you're planning to become a mother, talk to your physician about how much folic acid you need.

Preventing birth defects alone would make folic acid a nutritional superstar. But during the 1990s further research began to suggest that this versatile vitamin may play a critical role in combating the number one killer in Western civilization, heart disease. Studies involving large populations reveal that people with high levels of homocysteine have an increased risk for heart attacks. Scientists know that folic acid and vitamins B_6 and B_{12} clear homocysteine from the blood. Another large study found that women who consumed large amounts of folic acid and vitamin B_6—including many who got their big doses from supplements— had low rates of heart disease. Does that mean taking folic acid or B_6 pills prevents heart attacks? It might, but that theory needs to be confirmed with closer scientific scrutiny.

Several studies have also shown that people who consume lots of folic acid are less likely to develop certain cancers. More studies are necessary, though, to prove a cause and effect.

What else should I know about folic acid supplements?

Very high doses of folic acid may mask symptoms of vitamin B$_{12}$ deficiency, which can cause a serious form of anemia.

A balanced diet provides plenty of folic acid. But since many Americans steer clear of leafy greens and other healthful foods that are rich in folic acid, a little insurance may not be a bad idea—and you can get a full day's dose of this important nutrient from a multivitamin.

Bottom line

Women should talk to a physician about taking folic acid *before* deciding to get pregnant. Some evidence suggests that the vitamin may help reduce the risk of cardiovascular disease, especially if you have high homocysteine levels; ask your primary-care physician about having your homocysteine levels measured.

GARLIC

Scientific name: *Allium sativum*

What is it?

An indispensable and piquant ingredient in many culinary traditions, the so-called stinking rose has also played an important role in folk medicine for centuries. Today, garlic cloves are dried and processed to produce a powder, which is packaged and sold in tablet or capsule form. Garlic oil preparations are available, too.

Why do some people take garlic supplements?

Over the years, garlic has been used for a long list of purposes—everything from relieving sinus congestion to treating snakebites. But most

Americans who take garlic supplements do so to lower their risk of heart disease, specifically to lower blood pressure and cholesterol.

Do they work?

Although garlic is one of the most widely studied of all medicinal herbs, there's no consensus as to whether taking the supplements can diminish the risk of a heart attack. Results from studies are contradictory: Some research papers show that they might, while others suggest that garlic doesn't lower blood pressure or improve cholesterol levels. However, the trend in studies performed in recent years appears to suggest that garlic does not lower cholesterol—both pills and oil extracts have flunked in several high-profile experiments. Furthermore, even defenders of garlic supplements will concede that if the herb works at all, the effect is rather modest. That's especially true when you compare garlic with prescription drugs used to treat hypertension and cholesterol problems.

What else should I know about garlic supplements?

For one thing, they don't contain any constituents you won't find in fresh garlic. A standard daily dose of 900 milligrams of dried garlic in a capsule or tablet equals roughly a half to one whole clove. As lovers of certain spicy foods know too well, garlic can leave you scrambling for the mouthwash after dinner. Likewise, heavy use of garlic supplements can taint your breath and even give your perspiration a foul odor. (Deodorized pills are available, however.) Some people who use garlic supplements also complain of stomach upset and other minor complaints.

Garlic supplements may exaggerate the effects of blood-thinning medications, such as aspirin or warfarin. Levels of these medications, which prevent blood from clotting, need to be carefully regulated; too much may cause potentially deadly bleeding, while too little could result in a blood clot. Many dietary supplements have the potential to interfere with this balance, which alone is a good reason to discuss their use with a physician. Garlic supplements may also interfere with drugs prescribed to diabetics for the control of blood sugar levels.

Bottom line

People with high blood pressure and cholesterol problems should not trust a product with a questionable track record that causes bad breath. Instead, talk to a physician about well-tested medications that are safe, effective, and don't require breath mints.

GINGER

Scientific name: *Zingiber officinale*

What is it?

The same spice that adds a peppery sweetness to many savory dishes, to say nothing of gingerbread and ginger ale, also has a long history as medicine. The fresh gnarly-looking roots sold at your local grocery are usually imported from Jamaica, although ginger is also grown in Africa and Asia. The dried and powdered roots are used to flavor teas and produce dietary supplements in many forms, including capsules, candies and chewable wafers, and liquid extract.

Why do some people take ginger supplements?

Although it's considered an all-purpose remedy in traditional Chinese and Indian medicine, ginger is most often used today to prevent and treat upset stomachs. In particular, many users swallow some ginger before setting sail to avoid motion sickness.

To a lesser degree, ginger is also used for some other conditions, including rheumatoid arthritis and heart disease.

Do they work?

Ginger may help soothe a roiling stomach on the high seas, though a few more positive studies would bolster the somewhat uncertain case for this use. One study found that Danish naval cadets who took a prevoyage dose of ginger (1 gram) were less likely to vomit or break into cold sweats. In another experiment, three dozen American college students who said they became seasick easily volunteered to be strapped into a special chair that tilted and rotated rapidly for six minutes. Some of the students were given ginger capsules, while others received either Dramamine or dummy pills. No one in the Dramamine or dummy-pill groups lasted the whole six minutes, but half the students in the ginger group stuck it out. On average, students in the ginger group stayed in the chair 36 percent longer than those who took Dramamine.

However, both fresh ginger and ginger supplements failed to prevent motion sickness in a similar experiment in 1991. Meanwhile, ginger hasn't always fared well in other studies of its role in calming other varieties of unsettled stomachs. For instance, doctors who've tried giving ginger pills to patients as a way to prevent postoperative nausea and vomiting have come away with inconsistent results.

Some intriguing research hints that ginger may help relieve the pain associated with rheumatoid arthritis, but much more study is needed. Other therapeutic uses of ginger have even less scientific support.

What else should I know about ginger supplements?

Few side effects have been linked to ginger, though there's little information about people who have taken supplements containing the powdered herb for long periods. High doses of ginger might interfere with blood-thinning drugs such as warfarin, as well as medications that control blood sugar in diabetics. According to some reports, lab studies suggest that the herb may cause mutations in human cells, which may make it unadvisable for pregnant women to use ginger.

Bottom line

Fresh ginger is inexpensive and easy to find. There's probably no harm in trying a bite-size piece to prevent or quell stomach upset, though there's no guarantee that it will work. Ginger supplements haven't been proven safe and effective to use. If you suffer from bouts of nausea, see a physician.

GINKGO

Scientific name: *Ginkgo biloba*

What is it?

The oldest living species of tree, the ginkgo is native to Asia, but also grows in other parts of the world. The fan-shaped leaves have been used in folk medicine for at least five thousand years. Today, they're dried and usually sold in pill form. Ginkgo biloba extract is one of the most widely prescribed medications in Europe, where in most countries it is regarded as a drug.

Why do some people take ginkgo supplements?

Ginkgo is best known as a memory booster, making it particularly attractive to baby boomers and senior citizens struggling with their ability to recall names and facts. The herb is also being studied as an alternative therapy for Alzheimer's disease and other forms of dementia (the loss of intellectual faculties such as memory, concentration, and judgment). Thanks in large part to the way ginkgo is marketed in this country, many Americans take the herb as a kind of "smart pill," believing it will "improve mental performance," as one leading brand claims.

Ginkgo has garnered a reputation for treating and preventing other conditions, among them circulation problems and erectile dysfunction.

Do they work?

There is some evidence that ginkgo may slow mental deterioration among people with dementia. For instance, a 1997 study in the *Journal of the American Medical Association* found that patients with mild to severe Alzheimer's disease remained stable if they took 120 milligrams of ginkgo a day. Meanwhile, the mental health of a similar group of patients who didn't take the herb worsened. A few other studies, most of them small, also suggest that the symptoms of Alzheimer's disease may respond to doses of ginkgo, though further research is needed. (The National Institutes of Health is presently sponsoring a long-term study of the effectiveness of ginkgo for preventing dementia, although the results won't be known until at least 2006.)

If you don't have Alzheimer's disease or any other form of dementia, there's not much reason to think that ginkgo will improve your memory—help you remember your spouse's birthday or the name of your fifth grade math teacher, for instance. Everyday forgetfulness is probably unrelated to the devastating loss of memory associated with various forms of dementia. Although some small studies have shown that people who take ginkgo improve certain aspects of their memory—such as remembering lists of numbers—that doesn't mean taking the herb every day will help you find your keys. The neurological processes involved in recalling lists of numbers may be distinct from those used to recall where you left an object earlier in the day. The fact is, no one can be sure whether ginkgo helps any type of everyday memory, since its role for that purpose in healthy people hasn't been adequately studied. Likewise, there's no solid research to confirm the suggestion that the herb can make you smarter or better able to concentrate.

Scientists do know that ginkgo has measurable biological effects in humans, however. For instance, it contains antioxidants, which protect arteries and cells, and appears to prevent sticky substances in the blood called platelets from forming clots. Ginkgo also causes blood vessels to dilate, which is why the herb has been studied for use in treating problems such as intermittent claudication, a condition characterized by pain and fatigue in the legs due to lack of blood flow. Unfortunately, the results of studies involving patients with this particular circulatory problem have been inconsistent.

Some psychiatrists recommend ginkgo to both male and female patients suffering from loss of sexual desire or potency brought on as a side effect of certain antidepressants. However, the evidence for ginkgo's role as an aphrodisiac is weak.

What else should I know about ginkgo supplements?

As mentioned, ginkgo may open blood vessels. If you're taking any form of anticoagulant medicine, such as aspirin or warfarin, adding this herb could produce internal bleeding. In fact, there has been at least one report of bleeding in the brain in one ginkgo user. Side effects associated with ginkgo are rare and usually limited to mild gastrointestinal problems.

Bottom line

Ginkgo appears to contain a drug (or drugs) that may affect how the brain functions in people with some conditions. But the herb's true benefits and safety won't be known until it undergoes more study. If you're having trouble remembering things, consider seeing a physician. Memory loss can be a symptom of depression or other conditions.

GINSENG

Scientific name: *Panax ginseng*, a general name for products labeled as Asian ginseng, Chinese ginseng, Korean ginseng, and American ginseng, although the latter is sometimes specified as *P. quinquefolius*
Not to be confused with Siberian ginseng (also known as pseudo-ginseng)

What is it?

Ginseng has been one of the most important herbs in Chinese medicine for over four thousand years. The American and Asian varieties of this modest plant are closely related. Ginseng grows wild throughout parts of the eastern United States and Canada, though the herb found in most products sold in this country is imported from commercial farms in Korea. (In an ironic twist, much of the ginseng grown by American farmers is exported to the Far East.) The roots of the ginseng plant are dried to produce an extract used in capsules, powders, liquid extracts, teas, and even soft drinks.

Why do some people take ginseng supplements?

In the United States, many consumers think of this herb as a caffeine-free source of vitality and energy. Traditional Chinese healers believe that American and Asian ginseng have distinct medical properties from each other and recommend them for different conditions. The Asian variety, in particular, is considered an all-purpose health tonic. Ginseng is sometimes referred to as an adaptogen, which is a term used by some proponents of natural medicines for a substance that allegedly helps the body cope with all forms of physical and mental stress.

Do they work?

There's little solid science to support the belief that this herb boosts energy and endurance. In some studies conducted overseas, athletes have improved their aerobic capacity (a standard measurement of physical fitness) while training if they took ginseng supplements. But most of these studies were seriously flawed. Some failed to compare the athletes taking ginseng with other athletes who didn't take the herb. Others simply involved too few people to draw firm conclusions.

As ginseng became popular in the United States—sales increased about 400 percent during the 1990s—researchers here took an interest in exploring claims that it improved athletic performance and physical stamina. The results of their studies have been disappointing, for the most part. For example, trials conducted at Louisiana State University and Wayne State University found that people who took ginseng supplements for several weeks weren't able to run any faster or longer than people who didn't. As for nonathletes, it's probably impossible to say whether ginseng "restores" or "reinvigorates" a fatigued body, since these vague claims are difficult to measure.

Few doctors or scientists in the United States believe in the concept of adaptogens, since it evolved from anecdotal reports, not experimental science. Studies of ginseng's role in improving immune function and preventing cancer have largely been limited to animals. Ginseng may one day prove beneficial for people with non-insulin-dependent diabetes mellitus. A recent study found that diabetics were better able to control blood sugar levels while taking ginseng supplements, though more research is necessary to confirm a role for the herb in treating the symptoms of this common disease.

In some studies ginseng has demonstrated an estrogen-like effect, but whether the herb mimics hormones in humans isn't known.

What else should I know about ginseng supplements?

Although believed to be reasonably safe, ginseng may cause side effects when taken in high doses or over a long term, including elevated blood pressure, nervousness, insomnia, diarrhea, and vaginal bleeding. Pregnant women should avoid ginseng, as should anyone taking blood-thinning drugs such as warfarin and aspirin, MAO inhibitors (a class of antidepressant), or medications that control blood sugar (which are prescribed to diabetics). In fact, if you're given a prescription for any drug, tell your doctor if you're taking ginseng.

Siberian ginseng (see page 176) belongs to the same plant family as the American and Asian varieties, but it has different chemical properties and should not be considered interchangeable.

Bottom line

Although it's clear that ginseng may have a variety of druglike effects, there's little reliable research to suggest that this herb offers important health benefits and is safe to use.

Ginseng supplements are expensive to produce, which may lead some manufacturers to skimp. ConsumerLab.com tested twenty-two brands of Asian and American ginseng and found that seven contained less active ingredient than the manufacturer stated on the label. Worse, eight of the products contained unacceptably high levels of pesticides.

GLUCOSAMINE

Pronounced "glue-CO-suh-meen"

What is it?

Glucosamine is a substance that plays an important role in the creation of body tissue, including cartilage, the smooth lining on the surface of joints. It's also found in the stuff that makes crab and lobster shells hard, known as chitin (pronounced "KITE-in"). Shells from crustaceans and other spineless sea creatures are collected and ground up for their chitin, from which glucosamine is extracted for use in dietary supplements. (Interestingly, chitin is also the raw material for a popular weight-loss supplement known as chitosan—see page 55) Glucosamine, which is sold in pill form, can also be synthetically produced.

Why do some people take glucosamine supplements?

To relieve the pain and stiffness associated with osteoarthritis, the most common joint disorder. As you age, cartilage wears away. The friction that occurs as joint bones rub together causes aches and limits flexibility. Injuries and certain diseases or infections can also bring on osteoarthritis. In theory, glucosamine supplements act like building blocks, helping to restore lost cartilage.

Glucosamine is often sold in combination with another supplement, chondroitin (see page 58). Glucosamine first gained popularity in Europe in the early 1980s. Along with chondroitin, it caught on in the United States after the publication of several books touting their benefits, and following a reasonably enthusiastic recommendation from *New York Times* health writer Jane E. Brody.

Do they work?

A study funded by the National Institutes of Health determined that preparations containing glucosamine and/or chondroitin may provide modest relief from arthritis pain. The authors analyzed fifteen previous studies involving the supplements and found that, while some of the research was marred by scientific bias and design flaws, the overall weight of the evidence suggests that these natural joint-pain relievers might ease osteoarthritis pain. Since these studies also suggest that glucosamine is virtually free of side effects, this may be good news for arthritis sufferers, many of whom rely on over-the-counter and prescription NSAIDs (nonsteroidal anti-inflammatory drugs), which can cause nausea and stomach ulcers. However, more research is necessary to expand our understanding of glucosamine—particularly whether it's safe to use over long periods and as effective a pain reliever as NSAIDs.

What else should I know about glucosamine supplements?

If glucosamine works at all, you may need to take it for several months before feeling any benefit, according to past studies. As mentioned, glucosamine is often teamed with chondroitin, but the supplements are also available separately; some studies show that the latter is an effective treatment by itself. A new variety of prescription NSAIDs, known as COX-2 inhibitors, are believed to cause fewer gastrointestinal problems than older drugs.

If you have recurrent joint pain, see a physician. Although osteoarthritis is often the culprit, aching joints can be caused by rheumatoid arthritis (which occurs when the immune system attacks body tissue), other diseases, or injuries.

Bottom line

Studies suggest that glucosamine may be an effective treatment for osteoarthritis, but more research is needed before it's routinely recommended. If you have chronic joint pain, see a physician.

GOLDENSEAL

Scientific name: *Hydrastis canadensis*

What is it?

This perennial plant grows in forests across North America, although over-harvesting has led to shortages in some regions. Cherokee Indians and other tribes used goldenseal as an eyewash and for cleaning wounds. It eventually became a common ingredient in popular health tonics peddled in the early 1900s. The dried roots are usually sold as teas or packaged in capsules.

Why do some people take goldenseal supplements?

It's often paired with echinacea (see page 72) for battling the common cold and flu. Goldenseal is also used to treat a variety of familiar conditions, including sore throats, diarrhea, and bladder infections.

Do they work?

It's impossible to say. Although many proponents of natural medicine consider goldenseal an essential medicine, modern scientists have hardly studied this herb. Package labels often hint that consuming goldenseal will strengthen your immune system. Although lab rats fed goldenseal produce greater numbers of infection-fighting antibodies, there's no research suggesting it has a similar effect in humans.

Goldenseal contains an alkaloid known as berberine, which has been used on occasion to treat diarrhea. A few studies show that berberine supplements may help reduce stool volume, but only in people with very serious diarrhea caused by food poisoning—who should be under the care of a physician. Berberine has also been shown to fight infection-causing organisms in the laboratory, but there's no proof that it acts like an antibiotic in humans.

What else should I know about goldenseal supplements?

High doses may cause a long list of side effects, including elevated blood pressure, nausea, and vomiting. High doses have also been reported to cause convulsions and difficulty in breathing. Goldenseal may interfere with heparin, a drug used to treat blood clots, and should be avoided by pregnant women.

Bottom line

Goldenseal appears to contain druglike chemicals that may improve the symptoms of diarrhea in some cases. However, these active substances may also cause significant side effects. Don't self-treat persistent or excessive diarrhea; see a physician instead.

GRAPE SEED EXTRACT

What is it?

When vintners crush grapes to make wine, they're left with stems, skins, and seeds. The latter—particularly from red grapes—can be processed to make cooking oil, as well as this dietary supplement, which is typically sold in tablet or capsule form. Grape seeds contain high levels of vitamin-like chemicals known as flavonoids, which are found in many fruits, vegetables, grains, and nuts. One role flavonoids play is to act as an antioxidant, soaking up naturally occurring substances in the body known as free radicals that damage arteries and may be involved in the formation of cancer cells. Grape seed extract is commonly sold in capsules. (Some flavonoids act like estrogens; read how that may affect your health in the separate entry for soy, page 178.)

Why do some people take grape seed extract supplements?

As antioxidants go, grape seed extract is believed to be quite potent; proponents often tout that it's "fifty times stronger than vitamin E and twenty times stronger than vitamin C." The supplements are sometimes pitched to consumers who don't drink alcohol, but want the heart-healthy benefits of wine.

Do they work?

There's growing scientific interest in grape seed extract, but it's too soon to say that the supplement can reduce your risk of having a heart attack or developing cancer. For example, rabbits fed a high-cholesterol diet are less likely to develop hardening of the arteries if they're also given extract of grape seed. Likewise, a British study found that antioxidant activity increased in the blood of humans who took 300 milligrams of grape seed extract daily. But well-designed trials, comparing the outcomes of people who take grape seed extract with others who don't, are needed before this supplement earns a place in the arsenal for preventing cardiovascular disease.

Although a few studies have found that the active substances in grape seed slow the growth of tumor cells in test tubes, it's still premature to call grape seed extract a cancer fighter. Some studies suggest that grape seed extract may improve circulation in people who have a condition called venous insufficiency, in which blood flow from the legs back to the trunk slows down. But the research is preliminary; more rigorous study is needed to determine whether these supplements aid circulatory problems. (See separate entry for pycnogenol, page 156.)

What else should I know about grape seed extract supplements?

Grape seed extract doesn't appear to cause any significant side effects, though more study is needed to better understand how this herb works.

As mentioned, grape seed extract is often considered interchangeable with pycnogenol (see page 156), though neither supplement has been adequately tested in humans. Flavonoids may be important to human health, but a diet that's rich in fruit, vegetables, nuts, and grains provides all the average person needs.

Bottom line

Interest in grape seed extract is based largely on its role as an antioxidant. It's worth noting, however, that studies have failed to show that better-known antioxidants, such as beta carotene, prevent cancer or heart disease. A qualified physician can discuss diet changes and other ways you can reduce your risk of heart disease and cancer.

GREEN TEA EXTRACT

Scientific name: *Camellia sinensis*

What is it?

After water, tea may be the most frequently sipped beverage in the world. Green and black tea leaves come from the same species of evergreen tree, *Camellia sinensis*. Black tea, the variety commonly consumed in the West, is made from leaves that are vigorously rolled, which releases an enzyme that gives them deep color and flavor. Green tea, which is popular in Asia and parts of Africa, is made from leaves that are gently processed. (A third variety, oolong, is a cross between the two.) Green tea is now sold in most supermarkets; the extract is derived from dried leaves and usually sold in capsule form.

Why do some people take green tea extract supplements?

Thanks to media reports about research (much of it preliminary) involving green tea, some concerned consumers take the capsules to reduce the risk of cancer and heart disease. Others, perhaps too tired to heat up a teapot, use green tea extract for the same reason they might brew a cup of Lipton—to perk up, combat mental fatigue, and sharpen their wits.

Do they work?

Rates of heart disease and certain cancers are low in Asian countries, where people drink lots of green tea. Although Asians may practice other healthy habits that protect them, some scientists believe that green tea contains valuable disease-fighting compounds. In particular, tea is a rich source of flavonoids, substances that are also abundant in fruits and vegetables. Test-tube studies show that tea flavonoids act as powerful antioxidants, neutralizing the dangerous activity of free radicals and preventing cholesterol from being oxidized (which stops it from clogging arteries).

Some research in animals suggests that green tea may slow the growth of tumors and cut the risk of heart disease. Much remains to be learned about the effect of green tea in humans, however. After all, not all studies have found that tea drinkers are healthier than other people. For example, in 2001, Japanese researchers reported in the *New England Journal of Medicine* that drinking a lot of green tea—as much as five cups a day—doesn't seem to reduce the risk of stomach cancer. More important, researchers need to rule out the possibility that green tea lovers have some other habit that protects them from disease.

Scientists are considering green tea extract for other therapeutic purposes. Weight loss is one. Swiss researchers recently found that men who took green tea extract burned more calories than men who didn't, a difference not explained by the caffeine content of the extract. However, more study is needed to confirm green tea's role as a slimming supplement. Could sipping tea keep you out of the dentist's chair? Some research hints that the oolong variety may prevent tooth decay, but more studies are needed.

A final note or two. Green tea extract, like tea itself, contains caffeine. Research shows that small amounts of caffeine can increase alertness and the ability to process information (while too much caffeine can have unpleasant side effects—see below). Many studies performed on green tea have involved the beverage. A study showing that tea drinking may have health benefits isn't necessarily an endorsement for tea-derived pill extracts. Supplement companies may inadvertently remove an important compound when processing tea leaves.

What else should I know about green tea extract supplements?

As mentioned, green tea extract contains caffeine, which can cause irritability and insomnia in high doses. Talk to a physician before taking any dietary supplement that contains caffeine, since high doses of the substance can cause adverse effects on the brain and cardiovascular system. (Caffeine-free green tea extract is available, however.)

Bottom line

More studies are needed to determine whether there's a role for green tea in fighting disease. Meanwhile, talk to your physician about ways you can reduce the risk of heart disease and cancer, including eating a healthy diet, exercising, and controlling high blood pressure and cholesterol, if needed.

GUARANA

Scientific name: *Paullinia cupana*

What is it?

This woody vine is native to Brazil's Amazon Basin, where natives chew guarana seeds or pound and dry them to produce an extract, which is used to make a beverage. As a dietary supplement, guarana seed extract is sold in pill form alone, but it's often blended with other herbs. Furthermore, soft drinks containing guarana have long been popular in Brazil and other parts of the world, and are now available in the United States.

Why do some people take guarana supplements?

For centuries, people of the Amazon have considered guarana an all-around health tonic and treatment for many conditions. Dietary supplements containing guarana are often promoted in this country as energy boosters and weight-loss aids.

Do they work?

Call it herbal espresso. Guarana may perk you up, but this exotic plant boosts energy because it contains a common drug: caffeine. Guarana seeds are a rich source of the stimulant. The label on one brand of guarana seed extract claims that two pills contain 90 milligrams of caffeine; that's slightly less than the amount in six ounces of brewed coffee, while a can of cola has 35–50 milligrams of caffeine.

There has been very little research on guarana in humans. No study has shown that the herb improves mental or physical performance—at least no more so than any other source of caffeine. Guarana is sometimes combined with the herb ephedra (see page 75) in weight-loss pills sold in health food stores and on the Internet. Although these preparations are advertised as "all-natural," it's important to know that ephedra contains an amphetamine-like drug, ephedrine. The Food and Drug Administration has compiled a long list of people who died or became seriously ill after using ephedra.

Claims that guarana releases its caffeine more gradually, making it a gentler stimulant than coffee or cola, aren't backed by solid studies. Some scientists believe that there are other potentially therapeutic substances in guarana, such as antioxidants. But whether they confer specific health benefits isn't known.

What else should I know about guarana supplements?

Caffeine is caffeine, whether it comes from your favorite beverage at Starbucks or a dietary supplement. Consume too much and you may develop anxiety, the jitters, and insomnia. Caffeine can also interact with some drugs, so beware if you're taking any form of medication. There's no reliable information about the long-term use of guarana.

Bottom line

Guarana contains caffeine, which causes unpleasant side effects in some users. Little is known about how other components in this herb affect health and whether they're safe for human consumption.

HAWTHORN

Scientific names: *Crataegus oxyacantha, C. laevigata*, and related species

What is it?

This family of shrubs and small trees grows in many parts of North America, as well as Europe and Asia. The leaves, fruits, flowers, and other parts of the hawthorn have been collected and dried for use as medicine since at least the first century A.D. Hawthorn tablets, capsules, and drops are sold in most health food stores.

Why do some people take hawthorn supplements?

This herb is frequently prescribed in Germany to patients with heart failure, which occurs when the heart can't pump blood fast enough to keep up with the body's demands. (Contrary to common belief, heart failure does not cause the heart to quit beating altogether, and can be treated.) Herbalists recommend hawthorn for the same condition in this country; it's also frequently blended with other herbs in so-called cardiovascular tonics.

Do they work?

Hawthorn appears to contain substances that act like standard heart medications known as ACE inhibitors, which are sometimes prescribed to people with heart failure. Research performed in Europe suggests that hawthorn may improve some symptoms in people with early-stage heart failure. One study found that patients taking 600 milligrams a day of hawthorn were able to exercise significantly more (when tested on bicycles) compared with patients given look-alike placebo pills.

But while hawthorn is one of the more closely studied herbs in Europe, there are still significant gaps in scientists' understanding of how it works. In particular, there's no solid evidence that it's as safe or effective as standard drug therapy used to treat heart failure in the United States. Furthermore, if hawthorn does indeed affect heart function, it shouldn't be used without the supervision of a qualified physician. Any additional benefits hawthorn may hold for the cardiovascular system are purely theoretical, since other uses haven't been well studied.

What else should I know about hawthorn supplements?

Use of this herb may make you sleepy and cause your blood pressure to dip. It could also cause your heart to beat irregularly. The consequences of long-term use aren't known. Hawthorn may exaggerate the effects of digoxin, a drug prescribed for some heart conditions, and interfere with the body's ability to absorb iron.

Bottom line

Prescription medications used to treat cardiovascular problems, including heart failure, have been studied extensively. Large-scale trials have shown that heart failure patients who take ACE inhibitors not only feel better, but they may also live longer. Far less is known about hawthorn's benefits, to say nothing of its long-term safety, in the treatment of this serious and complex medical condition.

HORSE CHESTNUT EXTRACT

What is it?

The family of shade trees known by the name horse chestnut grows in the United States and Europe. (In fact, they line the Champs-Élysées in Paris.) Sometimes known as the buckeye, this tree reaches heights up to 100 feet and produces mahogany-colored nuts, or seeds. The seeds are processed to produce horse chestnut extract, which in this country is usually sold in capsule form.

Why do some people take horse chestnut extract supplements?

Horse chestnut is one of the most widely prescribed herbs in Germany, where the government has approved its use for the treatment of circulatory problems in the leg veins, notably chronic venous insufficiency. This disease, which afflicts up to 15 percent of men and 25 percent of women in the United States, is characterized by pain, cramps, and swelling in the lower limbs and is often accompanied by varicose veins. Various herbal preparations containing horse chestnut extract are sold here, and promoted as treatments for leg vein disorders.

Do they work?

Horse chestnut has been studied primarily in Europe, where scientific standards of proof that a medicine works are less stringent than in the United States. However, a 1998 review of the existing research suggests that this herb may relieve swelling and other symptoms of chronic venous insufficiency. Doctors in the United States often recommend the use of compression stockings for this problem. A study published in *The Lancet*, a British medical journal, found that horse chestnut works about as well as compression hose, though the latter therapy provided faster relief.

There is no reliable evidence that taking horse chestnut will eliminate varicose veins or hemorrhoids, as is sometimes suggested by natural medicine proponents.

What else should I know about horse chestnut extract supplements?

Never consume unprocessed horse chestnut seeds or tea made from them; in its raw form, this herb can be poisonous. Manufacturers say they remove the toxins before processing horse chestnut extract, although—given the lack of oversight in the dietary supplements market—such claims can't be guaranteed. A small number of people who take the pills complain of itchy skin, nausea, headaches, and other side effects. It may not be safe to use any form of horse chestnut if you're taking anticoagulant medication (such as warfarin or aspirin); some reports suggest that this herb will interact with these drugs.

Many horse chestnut products are "standardized" to contain a specific amount of escin, the chemical some scientists theorize may relieve leg swelling.

Bottom line

Some studies suggest that this herb may reduce the symptoms of chronic venous insufficiency. But the substance or substances that provide this druglike effect may also have side effects. Unexplained swelling or pain in the legs may be a sign of a more serious condition, such as a blood clot, and warrant immediate medical attention.

INOSITOL

What is it?

Inositol is a form of sugar that's found in cell membranes and may play a part in the transmission of hormones and neurotransmitters between cells. It's often identified—erroneously—as a B vitamin. Unlike vitamins, inositol can be manufactured by the human body, though a balanced diet provides plenty of the substance, too. Breast milk is a rich source of inositol, as are beans, grains, and nuts, as well as meats and dairy products. As a dietary supplement, inositol is usually sold as tablets or as a powdered beverage.

Why do some people take inositol supplements?

Some supplement sellers claim that inositol is a "fat burner" that also helps lower cholesterol and stops hair loss. It has also been used experimentally for the treatment of some mental health conditions.

Do they work?

There is no solid scientific evidence that taking inositol supplements will reduce body fat or weight, lower cholesterol, or prevent baldness. The latter claim is a good example of how companies that market dietary supplements exaggerate and distort science for commercial gain. It appears to be based on studies of lab rats, which lose fur if they're fed a diet low in inositol. But no research has ever proven that humans who take high doses of inositol are less likely to lose their locks.

Inositol has been studied for use in conventional medicine, such as the treatment of premature infants. There has also been a small amount of research involving the use of inositol to treat several psychiatric conditions. According to some reports, patients diagnosed with depression often have low levels of inositol in their brains. One small trial found that these supplements improved mood better than placebo in depressed people, but those findings need to be replicated in a larger group. Other studies suggest that inositol doesn't enhance the effect of antidepressant drugs. Preliminary research suggests that inositol may have a role in the treatment of panic disorder and obsessive-compulsive disorder, though studies have been small and findings inconclusive.

What else should I know about inositol supplements?

The average person consumes about 1 gram of inositol each day from a typical diet. In studies of inositol, subjects are often given more than ten times that amount. No one knows whether such high doses are safe.

Bottom line

Too little is known about the safety and efficacy of inositol to recommend its general use.

IRON

What is it?

Iron is a mineral necessary to form hemoglobin, the pigment in red blood cells that carries oxygen to body tissue. It's also needed to produce myoglobin, which stores oxygen in muscles, as well as some enzymes.

Although the body recycles iron, you still need to consume some each day from the diet, which is why it's considered an "essential" mineral. Animal foods are the best sources, since they contain a form of iron (known as heme iron) that's more easily absorbed by the body. Some plant foods, such as legumes (especially soybeans) also contain moderate amounts of iron. (And the iron in all plants, known as nonheme, may be absorbed better if it's consumed at the same time as vitamin C.) In the United States, breakfast cereal, bread, pasta, and other grain foods are fortified with iron.

Iron supplements are usually sold in tablet form. Most multivitamins contain a day's worth of iron, too, unless their labels state otherwise.

Why do some people take iron supplements?

To prevent and treat anemia. Also to improve athletic performance, particularly in endurance sports, such as long-distance running.

Do they work?

Iron supplements are an effective treatment for anemia caused by low levels of this mineral. Iron deficiency is the most common cause of anemia among women of childbearing age in the United States. A poor diet, heavy menstruation (the most common cause in women), and conditions that cause blood loss or interfere with the body's ability to absorb iron can cause this form of anemia. Another common cause of iron deficiency, especially in men and postmenopausal women, is the loss of blood through the gastrointestinal tract from a tumor or ulcer. Blood in the stool is not always visible, but if you notice some, see a physician promptly.) The symptoms of iron-deficiency anemia include fatigue, anorexia, infections, and skin and stomach problems, among others. However, the condition can also be symptom-free.

Pregnant women also have an increased need for iron. Vegetarians who do not consume plenty of dairy products, legumes (particularly soybeans), and other nonmeat iron sources may become deficient. But iron supplements should be used only after consulting with a physician.

According to one estimate, 3–5 percent of U.S. women aged eighteen to forty-four suffer from iron-deficiency anemia. However, as many as 13 percent of American women may be moderately low in iron. Their blood levels haven't sunk enough to be considered anemic, but their stored iron is too low. This problem may be particularly common among younger women who are physically active, especially serious long-distance runners.

One small study found that women with moderate iron deficiency (but who were not anemic) developed greater endurance and more speed in a fifteen-kilometer cycling test after taking iron supplements for six weeks compared to women taking sugar pills. However, follow-up studies would be necessary to confirm that finding, and there's no reason to think that athletes who aren't iron deficient will benefit from upping their iron intake beyond the recommended daily allowance. In fact, excess iron can be toxic (see the next section).

What else should I know about iron supplements?

Some people who use iron supplements develop black stools. Large doses can cause upset stomach and other gastrointestinal problems.

About four of every thousand Americans inherit a condition called hemochromatosis, which can cause serious health problems if too much iron is consumed, including damage to the heart, liver, and pancreas, as well as arthritis and skin discoloration (that is, it turns gray). Which is all the more reason to talk to your doctor before taking iron supplements.

Bottom line

A balanced diet that satisfies the recommended daily allowances for vitamins and minerals provides plenty of iron for the average person. People who develop iron deficiency must be evaluated by a physician.

KAVA

Scientific name: *Piper methysticum*
Sometimes called cava, kava-kava, and other names

What is it?

Kava is a shrub that belongs to the pepper family and grows on Fiji, Tonga, and other islands in the South Pacific. The roots and underground stems of the plant are used to make a kind of cocktail that's gulped among friends, often in publike kava bars. The herbal beverage is also consumed as an accompaniment to island ceremonies. In the United States kava is most often sold in capsule form or as tea.

Why do some people take kava supplements?

To relieve stress and anxiety, as well as to treat insomnia. Kava tea is promoted as a relaxing nonalcoholic drink. Likewise, supplement companies sometimes portray the pills as all-natural—and hence, safer, it's suggested—narcotics. At least one web site compared kava to Valium, with no risk of side effects.

Do they work?

Kava has been the subject of many scientific studies, but none meets the strict standards used in the United States to confirm the safety and effectiveness of prescription and nonprescription drugs. However, a recent analysis of seven trials suggests that kava may provide relief for mild anxiety. Most of the studies were small, and used varying doses of the herbal extract. However, the research consistently showed that people gripped by anxiety felt better after taking kava supplements.

Kava extract has not been well studied for use as a sleep aid. While kava may have a druglike effect, no one knows whether it's as safe and effective as standard antianxiety medications or sleep aids. In a broader sense, scientists don't know how kava affects the body, particularly the brain (see next section for some important cautions).

What else should I know about kava supplements?

A few side effects have been reported with moderate use of kava, such as relatively rare cases of gastrointestinal upset and skin rashes. The herb may also react with some medications; for instance, it may intensify the sedating effects of Xanax.

Although it's often portrayed as a kind of harmless "happy herb," kava should not be taken lightly. Even at mild doses, it acts as a sedative, making driving inadvisable. In fact, there have been cases reported in California and Utah of motorists arrested for drunk driving—who, it turns out, were intoxicated on kava beverages, not booze. (By the way, kava isn't known for its great taste; in Tongan, the word means "bitter.")

Bottom line

Kava may be a brain-altering drug. If you're concerned about anxiety, talk to a physician. Treating anxiety, depression, or any other psychiatric condition is serious business. The wrong drug may cause dependence or worsen the condition (even increasing the risk of suicide).

KELP

Scientific name: various species from the order *Laminariales*
Also known as bladderwrack, brown algae

What is it?

Kelp is the common name for many different varieties of seaweed, often brown in color, found in cold seas around the world. Some species of these marine plants can grow to be over two hundred feet long. Kelp, like other seaweeds, is a rich source of iodine. It has been used to make fertilizer, automobile tires, and ice cream. Kelp pills and powders are sold at most health food stores.

Why do some people take kelp supplements?

Some sources, particularly websites that sell kelp, recommend the supplements for the treatment of hypothyroidism. Kelp is also suggested for many other conditions, including rheumatoid arthritis and multiple sclerosis, and is often sold alone or combined with other herbs as a weight-loss supplement.

Do they work?

There's no way of knowing whether kelp is a viable treatment for hypothyroidism, since the seaweed hasn't been well studied. But that seems beside the point, since using kelp supplements for any reason can't be recommended.

The thyroid regulates body metabolism—the rate at which you burn energy. Hypothyroidism results in an underactive thyroid. Kelp allegedly stimulates the thyroid because of its high iodine content. Iodine is a component of certain thyroid hormones. But attempting to alter levels of thyroid hormones with dietary supplements and without a doctor's supervision is dangerous. Not only is balancing hormones a delicate science, but the iodine content of kelp varies greatly, even within a given species—there's no guarantee you'll be getting an accurate dose.

The belief that kelp speeds weight loss is based on the idea that obesity is caused by an underactive thyroid. But eating too much and not exercising enough are the main causes of obesity, not underactive thyroids. Furthermore, there's no way to predict whether it will work or is safe to use, since so little is known about kelp's role as a diet aid and in treating other health conditions.

What else should I know about kelp supplements?

As mentioned, kelp supplements haven't been well studied, so it's impossible to vouch for their safety. Some kelp supplements may contain high levels of iodine, which would make them dangerous to use. Kelp may interfere with drugs intended to treat thyroid problems. Some people are allergic to iodine and there has been at least one report of a severe allergic reaction to kelp.

Bottom line

Too little is known about the safety and benefits (if there are any of the latter) of taking kelp supplements. Because they could contain high levels of iodine, these products may cause serious health hazards.

LECITHIN

Other name: phosphatidylcholine

What is it?

Lecithin is a type of fat that's found in the cell membranes of most plants and animals, including humans. Among other roles, lecithin is a component of the sheath that protects nerves. Egg yolks, corn, and soybeans are rich in lecithin. Lecithin is also a common ingredient in prepared foods, such as margarine, snack crackers, and chocolate. That's because it acts as an emulsifier—that is, it helps fats bind with other ingredients. Lecithin supplements are usually derived from soybean oil and sold as capsules, liquid, powder, and granules (which are sprinkled on food or dissolved in beverages).

Why do some people take lecithin supplements?

Ask a health food store clerk for a pill to help lower cholesterol and you may be directed to the lecithin shelf. A few other common claims about lecithin: it prevents gallstones, boosts memory, and wards off neurological diseases, such as Alzheimer's.

Do they work?

Lecithin's reputation for maintaining healthy cholesterol levels is based largely on the unproven theory that lecithin deficiency leads to high cholesterol. Studies showing that lecithin may benefit the heart are considered outdated and seriously flawed. Although too small to be conclusive, a more recent study found that taking 20 grams of lecithin each day failed to lower high cholesterol in twenty men.

Lecithin is a source of choline (see page 56), a brain chemical that may play a role in memory. Because choline is needed to produce the brain chemical acetylcholine, some scientists theorize that it may improve memory. One research group gave varying doses of lecithin (in the form of phosphatidylcholine) to eighty college students, then tested their ability to recall sets of nonsense syllables, such as RIX, VAY, and XEJ. The phosphatidylcholine appeared to significantly improve the students' powers of recall. However, the findings from one small study are not enough to call lecithin a magic memory booster; no other studies prove that these supplements banish everyday forgetfulness.

Most studies of lecithin for the treatment of Alzheimer's disease have been disappointing, showing that increasing intake with supplements does nothing to prevent or slow the progression of the debilitating condition. Likewise, there's no scientific rationale for taking lecithin pills or granules to dissolve gallstones.

What else should I know about lecithin supplements?

Taking lecithin supplements may cause minor gastrointestinal side effects, such as diarrhea or nausea.

Bottom line

There is too little evidence to recommend using lecithin supplements for any purpose.

LICORICE

Also known as glycyrrhiza and liquorice

What is it?

You probably know licorice as red or black candy twists, though you may be surprised to learn that many varieties sold in the United States actually contain little or no licorice (they're flavored with anise oil instead). The licorice plant grows in Asia and Mediterranean countries, and has been used as medicine for over four thousand years. Licorice roots are boiled to produce an extract that can be used to make a tea. The herb is also sold in other forms, notably capsules.

Why do some people take licorice supplements?

Traditional healers recommend licorice for a wide variety of conditions, particularly upper-respiratory complaints such as coughs, colds, and sore throats. It's also promoted as a treatment for ulcers.

Do they work?

Although licorice root contains a variety of chemicals that may have druglike effects, it's impossible to say whether this herb lives up to its billing. That's because licorice's role as a medicine has primarily been studied in humans for one condition, ulcers. Research dating back to the 1940s suggested that licorice extract was an effective treatment for gastric (or stomach) ulcers. Unfortunately, ulcer sufferers who used licorice often developed unpleasant side effects, such as severe swelling of the face and limbs.

Researchers subsequently created a modified version of the herb, known as deglycyrrhizinated licorice, or DGL, which was designed to reduce the risk of side effects. But DGL's value as an ulcer fighter is questionable. Results from several studies of patients with stomach and intestinal ulcers are inconclusive at best, with several large trials showing that DGL worked no better than sugar pills.

What else should I know before taking licorice supplements?

Licorice contains steroidlike substances that, in high doses, can wreak havoc on your health. For example, consuming lots of licorice—whether as an herb or in candy—may cause the body to retain sodium and lose potassium, which can lead to high blood pressure and hypokalemia, a condition that can cause abnormal heartbeat, weakness, and paralysis. (The DGL form of licorice is touted as less risky to use, but that hasn't been demonstrated in proper safety studies.) Licorice may also interfere with MAO inhibitors (a class of antidepressant) and certain immune-system drugs, as well as medications intended to regulate heart rhythm, electrolyte levels, and blood sugar.

According to a 1999 letter to the *New England Journal of Medicine*, young men who ate a modest amount of licorice root every day experienced significant drops in testosterone levels, which could lead to loss of libido and other problems. Other studies, including laboratory research by one of this book's authors (Robert S. DiPaola, M.D.), have revealed that licorice contains molecules that act like the hormone estrogen. Although more research is necessary, it appears as though these and other herbal estrogens may have an important impact on human health. (See separate entries for soy and PC-SPES, an herbal preparation that contains licorice, on pages 178 and 149, respectively).

If you think you may have an ulcer, or suffer from frequent gastrointestinal pain, see your physician. He or she can determine the cause of your symptoms and prescribe proper treatment. (Recurrent pain in the gut can be caused by many conditions, including cancer.)

Bottom line

There's currently no scientific evidence to recommend the use of licorice root. In fact, this herb may alter levels of certain electrolytes and hormones, causing serious side effects.

LUTEIN

Pronounced "LOO-teen"

What is it?

Lutein is one of the carotenoids, which is a group of substances necessary for the formation of vitamin A in the body. (Another carotenoid, beta carotene, is discussed on page 36.) Lutein is also a pigment, found in great concentrations in the retina. Lutein is plentiful in corn, spinach, kale, broccoli, oranges, grapes, zucchini, and other plant foods. Egg yolk is another rich source. Lutein supplements are usually sold as capsules.

Why do some people take lutein supplements?

To improve vision and protect the eyes from age-related diseases such as cataracts (a gradual clouding of the lens) and macular degeneration (the loss of important pigment in the retina). Over a million Americans have cataracts removed each year and macular degeneration is the leading causes of blindness among the elderly in this country.

Do they work?

The view of lutein's role in safeguarding eye health remains rather fuzzy. Some scientists theorize that it may protect the eyes in two ways. First, lutein is known to be an antioxidant, which means it disarms substances called free radicals that could harm healthy cells in the eye. Second, this nutrient may act as a filter, its pigment absorbing ultraviolet rays from the sun that could damage the eyes.

Researchers looking for a link between nutrition and vision have uncovered some tantalizing evidence about lutein. For example, two studies performed in the 1990s determined that people who consume large amounts of leafy green vegetables, such as spinach and broccoli, have a reduced risk for macular degeneration and cataracts. The authors of both scientific papers speculated that lutein may be one of the keys to sharp vision, along with a related carotenoid, zeaxanthin.

However, people who eat lots of vegetables may have other healthy habits that limit their risk for age-related eye diseases. For instance, they may be less likely to smoke tobacco, which could lower their risk of cataracts and macular degeneration. But although much remains to be learned about the role of this nutrient in protecting vision, it's important to note that very little research to date has involved lutein supplements. While there's a small amount of evidence to suggest that eating foods packed with this nutrient might promote healthy eyes, little is known about people who get their lutein from pills.

Lutein is also being studied for its potential roles in other areas of health. One study found that people who eat a diet that includes lots of leafy greens and other high-lutein foods have a reduced risk of colon cancer, though the benefit was modest.

What else should I know about lutein supplements?

It's hard to draw any conclusions about the safety of lutein supplements, since adequate studies haven't been performed. However, it's very difficult to overdose on spinach or broccoli.

Bottom line

There's little data to recommend the use of lutein pills. However, eating a diet that includes plenty of vegetables (especially foods that are rich in lutein and other carotenoids, such as spinach and broccoli) may improve health in a variety of ways.

LYSINE

Also called L-lysine

What is it?

Lysine is an amino acid, which is an organic compound that forms proteins—the building blocks of all life forms. You need to get lysine from food; meats, poultry, fish, and some legumes are good sources. Lysine supplements, sometimes identified as L-lysine, are sold as tablets and powders. The amino acid is also included in some lip balm formulas.

Why do some people use lysine supplements?

To treat recurrent herpes simplex infections, which cause cold sores on the mouth and genitals.

Do they work?

Scientists have shown that lysine can stop the herpes simplex virus from reproducing—in a test tube. In humans, lysine's usefulness in fighting this infection is less clear. A few small studies performed in the 1970s and 1980s found that herpes patients who took supplements containing the amino acid several times a day had fewer, less severe outbreaks than sufferers given empty placebo pills. However, critics of that research offered results from their own trials, in which lysine failed to stop skin from burning and blistering.

Who's right? It's impossible to say, although lysine may simply work for certain herpes sufferers and not others, for reasons that remain unknown. If it does work, some people may require very large doses of lysine to feel any benefit. The effectiveness of applying lysine formulas directly to affected areas, as with a lip balm, hasn't been adequately tested in humans.

Lysine is being investigated for other therapeutic uses, such as the prevention of heart disease, but there's no solid evidence to recommend it for this or any other purpose.

What else should I know about lysine supplements?

Some people who use lysine develop diarrhea and stomach cramps, which go away once they stop taking the supplement. There's not much known about the long-term use of lysine.

Not all sores in or around the mouth are caused by the herpes virus. Cold sores that can be traced to this virus usually take the form of blisters on the lip that eventually become ulcers or pits. Doctors can prescribe well-tested antiviral medications to treat herpes. Other viruses can cause mouth sores, as can various diseases, including cancer. Finally, about one person in five suffers from painful recurrent aphthous ulcers (often called canker sores).

Bottom line

Much more needs to be learned about the therapeutic value and safety of lysine. Cold sores can be serious business, and should be examined by a physician.

MAGNESIUM

What is it?

Magnesium is a mineral that plays several essential roles in the body. For example, it's needed to make muscles contract and to form various enzymes. Magnesium deficiency is rare, but can be caused by several conditions, including protracted diarrhea, alcoholism, disorders that interfere with the body's ability to absorb the mineral, and the use of diuretic drugs. (And to make matters worse, magnesium deficiency may lead to diminished levels of the minerals calcium and potassium.) Good food sources of magnesium include tofu, whole grains, nuts and seeds, leafy greens, and seafood. Because it neutralizes stomach acid, magnesium is a common ingredient in antacids. Magnesium is available in tablet form and is usually included in multivitamins and multiminerals.

Why do some people use magnesium supplements?

Some migraine sufferers take magnesium pills every day in hopes of preventing the attacks. The mineral is also occasionally used to battle chronic fatigue syndrome and attention deficit hyperactivity disorder, or ADHD.

Do they work?

Although the jury is still out, some studies suggest that magnesium may reduce migraine attacks. According to one theory, low magnesium levels in the brain cause blood vessels to constrict, triggering migraines. Although hard data are lacking, some headache specialists estimate that up to 50 percent of migraine sufferers may be deficient in magnesium.

Evidence from a few clinical trials shows that injections of the mineral can ease migraine pain. Some experts hold out hope that migraineurs who take magnesium pills can prevent the attacks from happening, or at least limit them. But so far the evidence is conflicting. A 1996 study found that a daily 600-milligram dose of magnesium appeared to reduce the frequency of migraines by 46 percent. Later, however, another team of researchers found that a similar (though slightly smaller) dose of magnesium offered no headache protection in a different group of migraineurs.

Some research hints that magnesium supplements may help people with chronic fatigue syndrome, though adequate testing for that purpose hasn't been performed. Other research suggests that there may be a link between magnesium deficiency and ADHD, but it's not yet clear that giving magnesium supplements to children or adults with the disorder will improve their ability to concentrate and focus.

What else should I know about magnesium supplements?

Too much magnesium can cause muscle weakness, diarrhea, and even heart problems. Although side effects occur primarily in people who abuse antacids and laxatives (particularly in people with kidney problems), don't take magnesium supplements to treat a medical condition without first talking to your physician.

Bottom line

More study is needed to understand magnesium's role in treating migraines. On the other hand, physicians can offer people who suffer from these severe headaches a variety of treatment options, which may include drug therapy (such as nonsteroidal anti-inflammatory agents, or NSAIDs, and ergotamine), if appropriate. Nonpharmacological approaches—learning to avoid circumstances that trigger migraines, for example—may also help.

MELATONIN

What is it?

Melatonin is a hormone produced by the pineal gland, a tiny, cone-shaped structure found deep in the recesses of your brain. Scientists believe that melatonin plays several roles in humans. One is to signal the body that it's time to get some sleep. Levels of this hormone increase dramatically in the evening, but as dawn approaches production slows to a trickle. Melatonin capsules and tablets are widely available, though the supplement is also sold in other forms, including liquid drops.

Why do some people take melatonin supplements?

In 1995, *Newsweek* named melatonin "Pill of the Year," contributing to a nationwide frenzy over the supplements that sent consumers flocking to health food stores. Much of the ensuing hype about melatonin focused on the hormone's alleged antiaging properties, as well as the possibility that it might prevent cancer and other diseases. However, melatonin is probably best known as a sleep aid. In particular, it's widely used to combat the effects of jet lag—the tiredness, mental fatigue, difficulty falling asleep, and general sense of malaise that often plague air travelers for a few days after passing through several time zones.

Do they work?

Taking melatonin when you buzz off to Bangkok or some other far-flung destination may help you beat the blahs, though whether or not this supplement actually prevents jet lag is still up in the air. In theory, melatonin supplements "reset" your internal biological clock, helping the body readjust to the schedule of light and darkness in a new time zone, allowing you to fall asleep and wake up along with the locals. Several studies in the late 1980s and early '90s found that passengers on transcontinental flights had briefer, milder symptoms of jet lag in the days after landing if they took melatonin.

However, these studies involved relatively small groups of subjects. A larger, more recent experiment examined the effects of melatonin on 257 Norwegian physicians who were flying home from a conference in New York City. On the day after returning home, doctors who took melatonin were just as likely to feel lousy as those who were given empty placebo pills.

Even if you assume that melatonin supplements can change the hour on your brain's sleep clock, there's still the problem of timing your intake of the pills. People who use melatonin to minimize the effects of jet lag frequently begin using the supplements a few days before traveling across time zones, to prepare their bodies in advance. But in a 1993 study, airline crew members who followed a similar schedule before flying from Los Angeles to Auckland, in New Zealand, ended up having worse jet lag than other crew members who started taking melatonin upon arrival. More worrisome still: the travelers who began using melatonin before arrival felt worse than fliers who didn't take the supplements at all. That could mean that mistiming melatonin doses does more harm than good.

Some studies have shown that an injection of melatonin will make you drowsy, though it's not altogether clear that taking the hormone orally has the same effect. Some scientific surveys, though not all, have found that levels of melatonin drop off with age. Promoters of melatonin supplements claim that the pills act like natural sleep aids, especially for the elderly. But the track record for melatonin supplements' value as a sedative is mixed. In some studies, it has appeared to help subjects doze off earlier, while in others people who took melatonin slept no better than usual. Larger trials are needed to clarify the hormone's usefulness in fighting insomnia.

Scientists have also looked at melatonin in the lab to determine whether it has a role in treating cancer. Although preliminary studies show some potential—it's possible, for instance, that the hormone weakens the defenses of tumor cells—more research is necessary.

What else should I know about melatonin supplements?

Proponents boast that melatonin doesn't cause the "hangover" associated with prescription medications, but some people who have used the supplements have complained of side effects such as headaches and unpleasant taste in the mouth. In general, not much is known about the long-term use of this hormone supplement.

Bottom line

Although studies of melatonin show some promise, it's not clear who—if anyone—might benefit from taking this supplement. Nor is much known about the safety of its long-term use. Insomnia can be a symptom of more serious disorders; if you struggle with sleep, talk to your doctor.

MILK THISTLE

Scientific name: *Silybum marianum*
Sometimes identified as silymarin

What is it?

Milk thistle is a weedy, purple-flowered plant that's related to the daisy and artichoke. It's native to Europe, though now it grows in other parts of the world, including the United States. Milk thistle's seedlike fruit has been used as medicine for over two thousand years; today it's processed in the form of capsules and liquid extract, as well as tea.

Why do some people take milk thistle supplements?

To protect the liver, especially from the damaging effects of alcohol. One of the liver's functions is to clear poisonous substances from the blood. But chronic heavy drinking can injure liver cells, interfering with this critical organ's ability to eliminate blood toxins. In Europe, milk thistle is also used to treat hepatitis and other liver diseases.

Do they work?

Milk thistle seeds contains several compounds known collectively as silymarin, which some scientists believe prevents toxins from entering liver cells, in addition to causing liver cells to regenerate. German health authorities approve of its use for treating liver damage, including cirrhosis, a condition often caused by alcohol abuse. However, there's still no conclusive proof that supplements containing silymarin are an effective treatment for this life-threatening disease. In a study of nearly a hundred Finnish soldiers, silymarin seemed to speed repair in livers damaged by alcohol abuse. In another study, cirrhosis patients who took the milk thistle derivative had a lower death rate than similar patients who didn't. Yet silymarin failed to help alcoholics in other trials—taking the herb didn't improve their liver function or make them live any longer.

These studies involved small groups of patients and used different endpoints—that is, they were designed to prove or disprove different things. Viewed as a group, they tell us very little about silymarin's liver benefits.

By the way, the most frequently studied component of milk thistle, silymarin, is reportedly found only in the seeds of this plant; preparations made with other parts may act differently in the human body.

What else should I know about milk thistle supplements?

No serious side effects have definitively been associated with the use of milk thistle; in fact, it was once considered food in some cultures. However, no one knows whether frequent use of silymarin supplements is safe, since no studies have been conducted to determine their therapeutic value or toxicity. According to some reports silymarin may lower blood glucose levels, so diabetics should be particularly careful with this herb.

Bottom line

Too little is known about milk thistle and its components to recommend their use for the treatment of liver problems linked to alcohol abuse or other causes. Furthermore, liver damage is just one aspect of alcohol abuse, which can lead to motor vehicle accidents and other often-deadly mishaps, as well as family and professional problems—none of which can be prevented by a dietary supplement.

MSM

Scientific name: methylsulfonylmethane

What is it?

MSM is a sulfur compound produced from lignin, which is a substance found in the cell walls of wood. To be more specific, MSM is derived from a by-product of paper manufacturing, known as dimethyl sulfoxide, or DMSO. Sound familiar? DMSO is sold as a pain reliever that's applied directly to the skin, though it has some serious drawbacks: DMSO causes a foul taste in the mouth and fishy body odor. MSM, however, is reportedly odorless.

Why do some people take MSM supplements?

Several popular books about MSM claim that the supplement provides relief for a long list of common painful conditions, including arthritis, chronic headaches and backaches, fibromyalgia, tendinitis and bursitis, carpal tunnel syndrome, temporomandibular joint disorder, and even heartburn. Some celebrities have publicly endorsed MSM.

Do they work?

Books about MSM are filled with anecdotes about people who put aside years of pain and suffering when they started taking these supplements. Some were able to reduce the amount of pain medication they had been using; others allegedly threw out their drug prescriptions altogether. Backers say that MSM works by inhibiting pain impulses on nerve fibers, decreasing inflammation, and other actions.

Unfortunately, it's impossible to say whether MSM is truly a miracle medicine, since there have been no large clinical trials to determine whether this sulfur compound relieves pain. One book claims that there have been over fifty-five thousand studies of DMSO, the compound from which MSM is derived. Yet, to date there's no published research that adequately compares people suffering from any given painful condition who took MSM with others who took placebo pills—the gold standard of scientific research. Until such studies are conducted, the medical community should view MSM with skepticism.

What else should I know about MSM supplements?

Supporters claim that MSM is safe, but little is known about the safety of this supplement.

Bottom line

Until MSM undergoes adequate testing in humans, no one can say for certain whether it's a safe and effective pain reliever.

MULTIMINERALS/TRACE MINERALS

What are they?

Although virtually all multivitamins contain essential minerals, these mineral-only tablets have become increasingly popular in recent years. Minerals are nonorganic compounds in food that are necessary for human health. Our bodies require relatively large amounts of some minerals, such as calcium and phosphorus. Other minerals, such as iron and copper, are only needed in tiny portions, which is why they're known as trace minerals or elements.

Multimineral and trace mineral supplements are sold as tablets, capsules, and liquids.

Why do some people take mineral supplements?

People who are the most enthusiastic about mineral supplements tend to fall into one of two camps. The first includes longevity seekers who believe that modern agricultural practices have depleted our food and water of important minerals. They claim that the very old ages reported in populations of people in the former Soviet Union and other parts of the world are explained by the mineral-rich drinking water and farm soil in those regions.

The other group includes athletes, especially bodybuilders, who believe that mineral supplements will increase physical power and endurance.

Do they work?

There is evidence that consuming certain individual minerals in the form of dietary supplements can have important health benefits. Iron or iodine deficiencies can be cleared up with mineral supplements. Taking calcium pills to strengthen bones is another good example. Other minerals are presently being studied to determine whether they, too, fight disease when consumed regularly in high doses. For instance, one ongoing trial is testing whether selenium supplements reduce a man's risk of prostate cancer.

However, the idea that you can avert disease and premature aging by overloading the body with minerals lacks scientific credibility. Other than the deficient conditions mentioned above, shortfalls of all other minerals in humans are uncommon. If you eat a balanced, healthy diet you probably get all the minerals your body needs. And even if you don't, most multivitamins provide at least some portion (often 100 percent) of the recommended daily intake for each mineral.

Some athletes use multiminerals or trace mineral supplements to build strength and endurance. But the evidence that these minerals provide any athletic advantage is weak, and high doses may be dangerous (see next section).

What else should I know about mineral supplements?

With minerals, as with vitamins, more is not always better—and potentially toxic. The risks associated with consuming excessive amounts of the various minerals are too numerous to list here, but can include heart rhythm disturbances, liver and nerve damage, and kidney failure.

Bottom line

Don't take multiminerals unless instructed by your physician. High doses of some minerals are toxic and potentially fatal.

MULTIVITAMINS

What are they?

Multivitamins were introduced in the 1940s and have become the best-selling category of dietary supplement in the United States. Virtually all brands of multivitamins contain a full slate of individual vitamins, which are organic compounds found in foods that have been identified as essential to human health, but which the body can't manufacture on its own in sufficient quantities. Most multivitamins also contain some or all of the essential minerals your body needs, too. (See the separate entry for multiminerals, page 138.)

Many manufacturers of multivitamins now offer special formulas that are designed to appeal to specific groups of consumers, such as men, women, seniors, and children (see separate entries for information on prenatal vitamins, page 154, and children's vitamins, page 53). Furthermore, some varieties of multivitamins contain added herbs and are marketed under names that suggest they'll improve some aspect of physical or mental health. For example, a multivitamin with added glucosamine may bear the words *joint health* on the label; if it contains Saint-John's-wort, the package might suggest that the pills will improve mood.

Most multivitamins are sold as tablets, though capsules and liquid form are available, too.

Why do some people take multivitamins?

As nutritional insurance. Most multivitamins provide at least a portion (and often 100 percent or more) of the recommended daily intake for all the vitamins and minerals.

Do they work?

Taking a daily multivitamin has been shown to increase levels of important disease-fighting nutrients in the body, particularly in older people, who may be deficient in some vitamins. Some research suggests that people who use multivitamins are healthier than nonusers. For instance, preliminary studies have detected lower rates of colon cancer among women who use multivitamins. However, it's not clear yet what that means. After all, it's possible that multivitamin users may have other habits that could protect them from cancer. They may be more likely to eat healthy foods or exercise frequently, for example.

Meanwhile, a recent population survey of over 1 million Americans found that people who pop a daily multivitamin are no more or less likely to die of heart disease. Overall cancer rates among the vitamin crowd weren't much different either, with one curious exception: Male cigarette smokers who used the pills were slightly *more* likely to develop cancer. Although not proven, that may have been due to the dose of beta carotene, which in other studies appeared to increase the risk of lung cancer in tobacco users.

So is a one-a-day habit worth the time and expense? The folic acid contained in every multivitamin may be worth the price alone, since this important B vitamin may decrease the risk of heart disease by lowering levels of a substance called homocysteine. (For more on folic acid's role in preventing heart attacks and even reducing the risk of cancer, see the separate entry on page 94.) A study of over fifteen thousand physicians should shed more light on the health benefits of popping a daily multivitamin, but its results won't be known for several years. Meanwhile, there's probably no harm in taking a multivitamin, and they could prove beneficial. (However, talk to your physician about the type of multivitamin you choose; some may contain excessive amounts of certain nutrients or untested herbs and other unsafe compounds.)

A multivitamin may be sound nutritional insurance. The fact remains that Americans don't eat right. The U.S. government has been telling us for years to eat three to five servings of vegetables per day, but fewer than one-third of us do so. (And that paltry figure is rather misleading, since French fries are counted as vegetables.) We eat even less fruit. Still, multivitamins do not replace a healthy diet. Scientists continue to discover micronutrients in foods that may prevent disease and improve health. And these phytochemicals are not typically found in multivitamins. An editorial in the *New England Journal of Medicine* sums up what may be the best advice succinctly: "Eat right *and* take a multivitamin."

What else should I know about multivitamins?

There's a reason they call them one-a-day pills; taking two or more multivitamins at once, to load up on nutrients, may be a bad idea. The body may absorb multivitamins better when they're taken with a meal. Beware of buzzwords on package labels, such as *time-release* and *chelated*—they have no proven value. Multivitamin formulas targeted at specific groups, such as men or women, often contain levels of certain vitamins or minerals that are higher than has been proven necessary for human health. What's more, there's little or no science to support the use of many herbs and other nonessential compounds added to some formulas—although some may carry risks.

Bottom line

Multivitamins are probably not harmful for most people and may provide some users a needed nutritional boost. However, popping a multivitamin is not a substitute for eating a balanced diet. Multivitamins that contain added herbs and compounds cost more, but may not provide any additional health benefits or be safe to use. Talk to your physician before adding a multivitamin to your regimen.

N-ACETYL CYSTEINE

Other names: acetylcysteine, NAC

What is it?

N-acetyl cysteine is a modified version of the amino acid cysteine, which is found in various proteins throughout the human body. Cysteine provides sulfur for several functions. As a drug, this amino acid is identified as acetylcysteine; the dietary supplement is usually labeled NAC and sold in tablet form.

Why do some people take NAC supplements?

Physicians rely on acetylcysteine as therapy for several conditions (described below). Some consumers—especially serious bodybuilders—use NAC in the belief that it acts as an antioxidant.

Do they work?

Doctors use acetylcysteine to treat patients who have overdosed on acetaminophen (the generic name for Tylenol). It also has demonstrated benefits

for people with acute and chronic bronchitis in some (but not all) studies; NAC may help break up mucus secretions. One study found that NAC may enhance the effect of drugs used to treat angina pectoris. However, when NAC is used in a hospital it's often in a form (such as intravenous) not available to consumers. More important, no one should ever attempt to self-treat any of these serious conditions with NAC or any other dietary supplement.

NAC supplements may increase levels of glutathione, a compound that plays an important role in muscle development. Heavy exercise appears to lower levels of glutathione in the body. One book extolling the virtues of bodybuilding supplements claims that taking NAC can boost glutathione levels up to 500 percent. It doesn't mention, however, that the evidence for this claim is a medical report involving a three-year-old girl who suffered from a rare condition that caused glutathione deficiency. Another study showing that NAC prevented muscle fatigue during exercise used an intravenous form of the amino acid. This supplement's role in building bigger muscles is based largely on theory, not on solid scientific evidence.

What else should I know about NAC supplements?

There are some well-established side effects associated with use of the prescription drug acetylcysteine, including the risk of vomiting, nausea, chills, coughing and wheezing, drowsiness, allergic reactions, and a runny nose. Some lab studies have shown that NAC interferes with the ability of chemotherapy to kill tumor cells, suggesting that this supplement may be inappropriate for cancer patients.

Bottom line

Leave the use of NAC (in the form of acetylcysteine) to physicians; this supplement may not be safe or effective for consumers to use without medical supervision.

NIACIN

Also known as vitamin B$_3$, niacinamide, and nicotinic acid

What is it?

Niacin is one of the B vitamins. Your body uses it to form enzymes that help convert carbohydrates, fats, and protein in food into energy. Niacin is also necessary to keep your nervous system running, to maintain smooth skin and a healthy digestive system, and to form sex hormones.

Most protein-rich foods are good sources of niacin, including poultry, fish, beef, peanut butter, and beans and other legumes. In pill form, niacin has an unusual dual citizenship—it's sold as both a dietary supplement *and* a prescription drug. That means you can walk into any store that sells dietary supplements and buy this vitamin without a prescription. Yet, niacin is also considered a drug, and a potent one at that.

Why do some people take niacin supplements?

Niacin is best known for its ability to lower cholesterol and other blood lipids that may cause cardiovascular disease. However, doctors prescribe high doses of this vitamin to treat a disease called pellagra, which is caused by a deficiency in the vitamin.

Do they work?

Yes, but there's a big catch. There's no question that niacin lowers cholesterol and provides other heart-healthy benefits. In a 1994 study of 136 people, high doses of the vitamin (up to 4.5 grams per day) lowered LDL cholesterol (the "bad" kind), though not as much as lovastatin, a commonly prescribed prescription drug. However, niacin also boosted HDL cholesterol (the "good" kind) more than four times higher than lovastatin.

So what's the catch? At the levels necessary to lower cholesterol, niacin can have striking side effects—some merely uncomfortable, others very serious. (Lovastatin and other so-called statin drugs, on the other hand, cause few side effects.) Keep reading and you'll see why no one should take niacin without the supervision of a physician.

What else should I know about niacin supplements?

A dose of niacin can leave you red in the face—literally. The skin of a niacin user typically flushes and turns prickly hot soon after taking the pills. The redness and heat usually subside within a few minutes, but some people find the sensation unpleasant and even embarrassing. High doses of niacin can also cause stomach upset. More important, they may cause liver damage, which is why anyone taking therapeutic doses of the vitamin must be regularly monitored by a physician. Furthermore, niacin supplements may raise blood levels of an amino acid called homocysteine, which could have the counterproductive effect of actually increasing the risk of heart disease (see separate entries for vitamin B$_6$ [page 192] and folate [page 94]).

So-called slow-release niacin is available in both supplement and drug form. In theory, these pills release niacin into the system more gradually, which is said to reduce skin flushing. However, not only have studies shown that flushing isn't entirely eliminated, but the drug form of slow-release niacin has been shown to be potentially toxic to the liver. Whether or not slow-release niacin supplements are safe or toxic isn't clear, which is all the more reason to talk to a physician before using this vitamin.

Before prescribing drugs or dietary supplements to lower cholesterol, doctors will often first recommend that a patient adopt a low-fat diet (with no more than 7–10 percent of calories coming from saturated fat) and get plenty of exercise. If cholesterol levels remain high, a physician will likely prescribe medication. Statin drugs (such as lovastatin) are often chosen over niacin and other interventions, since—as mentioned earlier—they're known to be effective and may cause fewer side effects.

Bottom line

Niacin is an excellent example of a dietary supplement with obvious druglike effects. It should be used with caution and only under the supervision of a physician.

PANTETHINE AND PANTOTHENIC ACID

Also known as vitamin B$_5$

What are they?

Pantothenic acid is one of the lesser-known B vitamins, but that doesn't mean it's not important to human health. It's necessary for the metabolism of nutrients, as well as the formation of certain hormones, neurotransmitters, and fatty acids.

Pantothenic (Greek for "from everywhere") acid is found in many different foods, so very few people become deficient in this vitamin. Nonetheless, pantothenic acid and one of its derivatives, pantethine, are sold as dietary supplements, typically in capsule form. Pantothenic acid is usually included in multivitamins, too.

Why do some people take pantethine and pantothenic acid supplements?

Pantethine supplements are used to lower blood levels of cholesterol and triglycerides, which are fatlike substances that increase the risk of heart attack. Pantothenic acid supplements are sometimes promoted as therapy for acne and arthritis. The vitamin is also often included in "stress-busting" and "energy-boosting" formulas.

Do they work?

A few studies suggest that large doses of pantethine may lower LDL ("bad") cholesterol and tryglicerides, while raising HDL ("good") cholesterol levels in people whose blood fats are out of balance. However, these studies involved small numbers of patients and need to be repeated with larger groups to know whether this B vitamin has any value in preventing heart disease. Furthermore, pantethine has a different chemical structure from pantothenic acid. The latter is cheaper and easier to find in health food stores, but no one knows whether it has any effect on cholesterol levels.

The evidence for pantothenic acid's therapeutic value in clearing up adolescent skin problems and relieving pain in aging joints is very limited. Likewise, there's no scientific grounding for claims that pantothenic acid will help you relax or make you exercise longer.

What else should I know about pantethine and pantothenic acid supplements?

Supplements of pantothenic acid and its derivative, pantethine, haven't been adequately studied for safety. Still, talk to a physician before taking any more than is found in a typical multivitamin. Keep in mind, too, that high cholesterol is serious business and that conventional medicine offers well-tested and proven medications for treating this condition.

Bottom line

Pantethine's role in lowering cholesterol is unclear (and there's no evidence to suggest that pantothenic acid will do the job). As part of a regular physical exam, have your cardiovascular risk factors evaluated by a physician. If you have elevated cholesterol, your physician may recommend exercise and a low-fat diet, which for some patients are enough to bring blood fats down to safe levels. If your cholesterol levels are very high or don't respond to lifestyle changes, your physician may prescribe medication.

PAPAYA AND PAPAIN

Scientific name: *Carica papaya*
Other names: papaw, pawpaw

What is it?

The juicy, yellow-fleshed papaya grows in tropical climates all over the world. Before it ripens, this fruit produces a milky sap that contains papain, an enzyme that breaks down protein molecules into amino acids. Papaya leaves contain a small amount of papain, too. In some culinary traditions, tough meat was wrapped in the leaves to make it less chewy; today, papain is an ingredient in some commercial meat tenderizers. As a dietary supplement, papaya and papain are commonly sold as capsules, tablets, and chewable mints, as well as blended with other natural enzymes. Some skin care products contain papaya and papain, too.

Why do some people take papaya and papain supplements?

To prevent and relieve indigestion. Papaya and papain are also used to treat other gastrointestinal problems, including constipation and worm infestation. They have also been recommended as complementary therapies for a long list of other conditions and diseases.

Do they work?

In theory, papain might act like pepsin and other digestive enzymes by helping to break down protein in the foods we eat. Proponents of papain and other enzyme supplements (see page 74) argue that undigested protein causes gastrointestinal discomfort, as well as other health problems, but there's no good evidence to back up such claims. In particular, there is no conclusive information in the Western medical literature about the use of papaya as treatment for the symptoms associated with indigestion or dyspepsia, which may include nonspecific abdominal pain, gas, bloating, and flatulence.

However, papaya *is* being studied for other therapeutic uses, such as wound healing and the treatment of spinal disk hernias. Still, commercial products (including skin creams and lotions) containing the fruit or its enzymes have no proven benefits. Even the herb-friendly German health authorities say there's not enough evidence to recommend papaya or papain for any health condition.

What else should I know about papaya and papain supplements?

Some people are allergic to papaya. There has been at least one reported case of papaya supplements inducing a skin rash. There is also some literature suggesting that papaya supplements may cause birth defects, which raises concerns about their use in pregnant women.

Bottom line

Further study is needed to understand the safety and effectiveness of these supplements.

Don't allow this skeptical view of dietary supplements that contain papaya and papain to steer you away from the fruit itself. Fresh papaya is not only delicious, but it's a nutrient powerhouse, packed with more than twice as much vitamin C and folate as a navel orange.

One medium navel orange contains about 75 milligrams of vitamin C and 44 micrograms of folic acid.

One medium papaya contains about 188 milligrams of vitamin C and 116 micrograms of folic acid.

Source: Bowes and Church's Food Values of Portions Commonly Used, 1998 edition

---

PC-SPES

What is it?

PC-SPES is a dietary supplement that contains a blend of eight herbs: chrysanthemum, isatis, licorice, *Ganoderma lucidum*, ginseng, *Rabdosia rubescens*, saw palmetto, and scullcap. PC-SPES is sold in capsule form.

Why do some people take PC-SPES?

PC-SPES is an abbreviation, of sorts. "PC" stands for "prostate cancer," while "SPES" is the Latin word for "hope." Accordingly, some patients with prostate cancer use PC-SPES in hopes that it will arrest the growth of their tumors. The use of PC-SPES for this purpose was promoted in a book titled *The Herbal Remedy for Prostate Cancer*.

Does it work?

Yes, but the benefits of PC-SPES must be balanced against its potential risks. Two studies, including one published in the *New England Journal of Medicine* and directed by a coauthor of this book (Robert S. DiPaola, M.D.), have shown that PC-SPES can shrink prostate tumors and control spread of the disease in most patients. Its effects can be sustained for extended periods—about three years, on average, in men who have not yet been treated with medical hormone therapy.

However, men who are receiving medical hormone therapy (such as Lupron, to lower testosterone levels) for their disease appear to gain little benefit from taking this herbal mix. (The same is true for men who undergo surgical castration.) One study showed that PC-SPES controlled prostate cancer in men for only sixteen weeks, on average, after standard medical hormone therapy failed. Furthermore, while hormone therapy carries a very small risk of side effects, the same does not appear to be true of PC-SPES. The *New England Journal of Medicine* study found that the herbs in PC-SPES contain potent forms of estrogen. Estrogen is the so-called female hormone. Therapeutic doses of estrogen can help control prostate cancer, though this form of treatment is seldom used, since it can have unpleasant and even fatal side effects. In the study, each of the eight men taking PC-SPES developed some of the same side effects that are associated with estrogen therapy, including breast tenderness and loss of libido. One man developed a blood clot.

PC-SPES, like estrogen therapy, may prove to have a role in the treatment of prostate cancer, since both forms of treatment can control growth of these tumors (though not permanently) in men with the disease after standard hormonal therapies fail. Researchers are comparing the benefits of PC-SPES with prescription estrogen.

What else should I know about PC-SPES?

PC-SPES's effects and toxicity are similar to prescription estrogen. Although its use cannot be recommended, if you choose to try PC-SPES, tell your physician immediately. The presence of these herbs can interfere with the accuracy of the PSA (prostate-specific antigen) blood test, which doctors use to screen healthy men for prostate cancer and monitor the status of tumors in men diagnosed with the disease.

As mentioned above, PC-SPES appears to cause similar side effects in men as those caused by estrogen therapy. They can include potentially lethal blood clots in the legs or lungs, impotence, and breast tenderness. PC-SPES is expensive; a ten-day supply costs about $100, which is not covered by most insurance plans. Finally, it's important to note that, like any therapy used to control prostate cancer, the effect of PC-SPES appears to be temporary.

Bottom line

PC-SPES contains potent plant estrogens that have the same effects—and side effects—as prescription estrogen pills (though the latter are better tested and controlled for quality). More research is needed to determine whether this herbal mix has other benefits and risks beyond those associated with estrogen. Safer, well-studied treatment options are available to men with prostate cancer. There are also promising interventions available to patients who enroll in clinical trials.

PHOSPHORUS

What is it?

Phosphorus is one of the most plentiful and important elements in the human body. It's found in every cell (mostly in the form of phosphate) and is necessary for the formation of DNA, your genetic blueprint. Phosphorus also plays a critical role in creating energy and combines with calcium to build molecules needed to make teeth and bones.

A wide variety of foods contain phosphorus, including beef, poultry, seafood, dairy products, eggs, grains, and legumes. It's also added to many processed foods. Because phosphorus is an unstable element, it must be combined with another element in dietary supplements. The word *phosphate* in a pill or powder indicates that it contains phosphorus.

Why do some people take phosphorus supplements?

This mineral is sometimes combined in supplements with calcium, which is widely used to strengthen bones. Some athletes take phosphorus in the belief that it will help them work out longer and harder. Phosphorus is also commonly used in the practice of homeopathy.

Do they work?

Phosphate deficiency is extremely rare. It can be caused by some medical conditions, such as certain parathyroid problems, and may occur in people who abuse alcohol or antacids that contain aluminum. However, most Americans consume plenty of phosphorus, more than their bodies can use. There's no reason to think anyone needs dietary supplements containing phosphorus in order to build stronger bones. In fact, if levels of this mineral rise too high, the body starts getting rid of phosphorus, which can weaken bones.

A limited amount of evidence suggests that phosphorus supplements may improve some aspects of athletic performance. In one study, for example, cyclists improved their times when given sodium phosphate supplements (1 gram, four times a day) for three days before a simulated forty-kilometer race. There are several theories as to why phosphorus may be a sports aid, though none has been proven. According to one, phosphorus acts as a buffer for the accumulation of lactic acid in muscles during exercise, which may contribute to fatigue. However, it's important to point out that the existing studies of phosphorus as a sports supplement involved just a handful of athletes; it's not clear whether this mineral is safe to use in large doses, or if it would confer similar benefits if tested in a larger number of athletes or in the general population.

What else should I know about phosphorus supplements?

No long-term studies have been done on people who use this mineral supplement. Very high doses could damage bones and possibly harden arteries, which in theory might cause heart attacks and strokes.

Bottom line

The theory that phosphorus improves performance in people engaged in endurance exercise has not been adequately studied. However, since excess phosphorus may cause health problems, talk to a physician before taking supplements that contain high doses of this mineral.

POTASSIUM

What is it?

Potassium is a mineral that helps regulate heart rhythm and keep the body's water levels in balance. It's also involved in the transmission of nerve signals and muscle contraction. Potassium is found in many foods; oranges and bananas are two good sources. Potassium supplements are available by prescription and over the counter; the mineral is also usually included in multivitamins.

Why do some people take potassium supplements?

Doctors prescribe potassium supplements to patients suffering from low levels of the mineral caused by a poor diet, illness, or the use of certain medications. There is currently some interest in using supplements of this mineral to treat high blood pressure, or hypertension. Potassium is also used to prevent leg cramps and fight fatigue.

Do they work?

To a patient suffering from very low levels of this critical mineral, potassium supplements can be lifesaving. Potassium may also play a role in controlling hypertension, though using oral supplements for this purpose without the close supervision of a physician is a bad idea.

A 1997 review of thirty-three studies in the *Journal of the American Medical Association* found that potassium supplements can significantly reduce elevated blood pressure, particularly in people who eat a high-sodium diet. However, potassium levels in the human body must be kept in careful balance. Excess potassium can cause deadly fluctuations in heart rhythm, especially in patients with kidney problems or heart disease, or who are taking drugs such as digoxin. The message is simple: Don't take potassium supplements unless a doctor prescribes them.

The various bodies that fund scientific research throughout the world have not made the study of leg cramp therapy a priority in recent years; there's little scientific evidence to support the use of potassium supplements for this nightly nuisance. Likewise, there's no reason to think extra potassium will give you an energy boost, unless you're deficient to begin with.

What else should I know about potassium supplements?

High doses of this mineral can be dangerous, even deadly, leading to cardiac arrest. Studies show that eating a diet rich in fruit, vegetables, and low-fat dairy products can help control high blood pressure, possibly due to the high potassium content of these foods.

If you're tormented by nightly leg cramps, see a physician. Not only are there medical treatments for leg cramps, but this annoying problem could be a symptom of a more serious condition, such as a blood clot.

Bottom line

High blood pressure is a leading risk factor for cardiovascular disease. Some studies suggest that potassium supplements may help control this condition, but—because of their potential for serious side effects—don't take them unless directed by your physician.

PRENATAL VITAMINS

Sometimes called maternity supplements

What are they?

Specially formulated multivitamins that contain higher doses of certain nutrients than you'll find in standard multivitamins. Prenatal vitamins may also contain medicinal herbs thought to provide relief for some symptoms related to pregnancy.

Why do some people take prenatal vitamins?

Pregnant women use these supplements to protect the health of their developing fetuses and make sure their own bodies are getting adequate nutrition.

Do they work?

When a woman becomes pregnant, her body's need for several vitamins and minerals increases. However, because pregnant women eat more food, getting most of those extra nutrients is usually not difficult, provided her diet is balanced. There are two important exceptions. Folate has been shown to reduce a fetus's risk for birth defects such as spina bifida; all women of childbearing age should ask their physicians how much of this valuable nutrient they should consume each day. Pregnant women may require 600 micrograms or more of folate per day, an amount that may be difficult to obtain from the daily diet. Ideally, women should begin increasing their folate intake before becoming pregnant.

Furthermore, the recommended daily allowance of iron for pregnant women is 30 milligrams of iron each day—twice as much as other women—to avoid becoming anemic. That's a lot of iron, when you consider that a good-sized steak has only 7–8 milligrams. To ensure that a pregnant woman consumes enough folate and iron, as well as all the other necessary nutrients, many physicians recommend taking prenatal vitamin formulas. Some doctors suggest that their patients use vitamin supplements that are available by prescription only. Before using an over-the-counter prenatal supplement, bring the bottle to a checkup for your doctor's approval.

Prenatal vitamins may eventually prove to offer other benefits. For example, one study found that low-income women who were given vitamin supplements during pregnancy were less likely to deliver premature, underweight babies. It's possible that the added vitamins made up for nutritional deficiencies in the women's diets.

What else should I know about prenatal vitamins?

Many pregnant women complain that swallowing a vitamin supplement makes them sick. Some brands of prenatal vitamins contain added herbs. Companies selling these products may insist they're safe, but since most herbs haven't been well studied—particularly for their potential effects on developing fetuses—such claims can't necessarily be trusted.

Bottom line

Any woman who could become pregnant should discuss her vitamin intake with a physician. The benefits of folate in preventing birth defects underscore this need. Prenatal vitamin supplements that contain herbs should be avoided.

PYCNOGENOL

Also known as pine bark extract
Pronounced "pik-NOJ-uh-nul"

What is it?

Pycnogenol is a fancy-sounding name for a dietary supplement made from something you might find in your backyard—but only if you live on the southwest coast of France. Pycnogenol is made from pine bark from the *Pinus maritima*, which grows only in that Mediterranean region. However, to complicate matters slightly, some makers of pycnogenol include grape seed extract (see page 108) in their preparations. Like grape seed extract, pycnogenol is a concentrated source of plant nutrients called flavonoids.

Why do some people use pycnogenol supplements?

Often described as an antiaging supplement, pycnogenol allegedly reduces the risk of a long list of diseases and conditions, many of which tend to worry people over forty. The list includes cardiovascular disease, hypertension, arthritis, cancer, and others. Some people use pycnogenol in the belief that it protects the skin from sun damage.

Do they work?

Lab studies show that pycnogenol is an aggressive antioxidant, scavenging naturally occurring free radicals that can damage arteries. But testing of the supplement in humans is in its infancy. In one study, smokers who took pycnogenol supplements experienced positive changes in their blood; the pine bark extract appeared to make substances called platelets less likely to clump together and form clots. Another study suggests that pycnogenol improves circulation in people suffering from venous insufficiency, in which blood flow from the legs back to the trunk slows down, causing pain and other symptoms. However, this modest amount of research, involving small groups of patients, doesn't allow us to make conclusions about pycnogenol's benefits for the general population.

Furthermore, no conclusive studies exist showing that humans reduce their risk for heart disease, or any disease, when they take pycnogenol. In fact, the Federal Trade Commission forced an Iowa-based company to quit claiming that its pycnogenol was an effective treatment for not only heart disease, but attention deficit/hyperactivity disorder, cancer, arthritis, diabetes, and multiple sclerosis. Although pycnogenol is an interesting supplement worthy of further study, there simply isn't enough evidence so far to make such claims.

What else should I know about pycnogenol supplements?

The safety of pycnogenol hasn't been adequately tested in humans.

Bottom line

Pycnogenol may show promise in the lab, but its benefits for human health haven't been adequately documented.

PYGEUM

Scientific name: *Pygeum africanum*
Sometimes called the African plum tree

What is it?

Pygeum africanum is a tall evergreen that grows in central and southern Africa. Pygeum (pronounced "pie-JEE-um") bark is used medicinally; the powdered extract is usually sold in capsule form, sometimes paired with saw palmetto (see page 171) or nettle root.

Why do some people take pygeum supplements?

To relieve the symptoms of an enlarged prostate. Also known as benign prostatic hypertrophy (BPH), this condition causes urinary problems in middle-aged and older men: a frequent need to void, often at night, and difficulty emptying one's bladder. Pygeum is a widely prescribed treatment for BPH in France and some other countries.

Do they work?

Pygeum hasn't been studied as extensively as another herb commonly used to treat BPH, saw palmetto. But a small body of research suggests that it may provide modest relief to men plagued by this frustrating problem. For example, one of the key symptoms of BPH is nocturia, or the frequent need to urinate at night, which disturbs sleep. A French study found that men with BPH who took pygeum reduced their late-night trips to the bathroom by one-third. The men also rated their quality of life as improved. A few other studies found that pygeum improves BPH symptoms, though only mildly, in some cases.

However, important questions about pygeum remain unanswered, particularly in regard to how it works. Some compounds that shrink the prostate may contain substances that act like the so-called female hormone, estrogen, which could produce unwanted side effects. (See the separate entry for PC-SPES, page 149, to read more about the potential benefits and risks associated with plant estrogens.) What's more, it's theoretically possible that pygeum could slow the detection of prostate cancer by interfering with the accuracy of the blood test used to screen for the disease, known as the prostate specific antigen (or PSA) test.

What else should I know about pygeum supplements?

Not much is known about the long-term use of this herb. Side effects aren't common, but it may cause stomach upset. Some people believe that using pygeum is unethical, since the *Pygeum africanum* is an endangered species.

Bottom line

More study is needed to understand how this herb works and whether it's safe. The symptoms of an enlarged prostate may mimic those of prostate cancer and other urological disorders—and should be checked out by a physician promptly.

PYRUVATE

What is it?

Pyruvate is a naturally occurring compound that's produced when your body metabolizes carbohydrates in food. It's also found in some foods, including red apples, red wine, and certain cheeses. Dietary supplements in capsule form are sold in health food stores.

Why do some people take pyruvate supplements?

Pyruvate is one of many dietary supplements that's touted as a weight-loss aid. It's also promoted as a strength and endurance booster for athletes.

Do they work?

If you're trying to lose a few pounds, pyruvate may help—but the expense and inconvenience of taking this supplement surely outweigh the very modest potential benefits. First, a bit of background. Pyruvate's reputation as a diet aid began to grow in the early and mid-1990s, with the publication of several studies of obese people who used the supplement. The results of one study in particular are often quoted by companies that sell pyruvate, who claim that it's clinically proven to increase weight loss by 37 percent.

That's technically correct, but highly misleading. First of all, that study involved only fourteen obese women who were sequestered on a diet ward in a hospital. Each day they were given doses of pyruvate several times larger than most manufacturers recommend using. The women did lose an average of thirteen pounds over three weeks, but a separate group of women who were given look-alike placebo pills also lost ten pounds, a difference of about one pound per week.

In a more recent study, pyruvate's pound-shedding potential appears more modest. A 1999 study divided twenty-six overweight people into two groups. One took 6 grams of pyruvate a day—which is the maximum dose most manufacturers suggest—while the other group took placebos. All subjects ate a modest diet and exercised regularly. After six weeks, the placebo group maintained the same weight, while members of the pyruvate group lost slightly more than 2.5 pounds, on average. That's a half pound per week—but at a cost that may exceed $100 a month.

Although these studies may appear promising, pyruvate needs to be tested in larger groups of subjects to understand its value as a diet aid. Scientists need to determine not only whether or not it increases weight loss, but also if it helps keep pounds off and can be used successfully by dieters outside a clinical setting. Finally, little is known about the risks associated with using pyruvate supplements.

There's no good evidence to support claims that pyruvate builds bigger muscles or improves athletic performance in any other way. In fact, a study of forty-two college football players found that taking high doses of pyruvate didn't increase strength.

What else should I know about pyruvate supplements?

There's not much information about side effects associated with low doses of pyruvate. In at least one study involving a liquid version of the supplement, some people who consumed large doses complained of gastrointestinal problems such as gas and diarrhea.

Bottom line

Losing weight can reduce your risk for several diseases. But the safety and value of pyruvate as a diet aid haven't been proven.

RED YEAST RICE

Scientific name: *Monascus purpureus*
Also known as Cholestin

What is it?

Fermented red yeast rice has been used in China since around A.D. 800 as a traditional medicine and to make marinade for pork ribs and duck. In the United States it's sold in capsule form.

Why do some people take red yeast rice supplements?

To lower cholesterol. According to the American Heart Association, about 100 million American adults have total blood cholesterol levels high enough to increase their risk for cardiovascular disease (generally considered to be 200 milligrams per deciliter [mg/dL]).

Do they work?

Probably, although red yeast rice represents one of the best examples of why consumers should regard dietary supplements just as seriously as prescription drugs. That's because it contains chemicals that are virtually identical to a category of drugs known as statins, which are widely prescribed for—what else?—lowering cholesterol.

It comes as no surprise, then, that a study published in the *American Journal of Clinical Nutrition* in 1999 found that the red yeast rice capsules sold under the name Cholestin lower total cholesterol. People in the study took 2.4 grams of Cholestin every day for eight weeks. By the end, their levels had dropped on average about 18 percent, from 254 mg/dL to 208 mg/dL. As far as herbal therapies are concerned, that's an impressive reduction. Yet, in this study, Cholestin did not appear to be as effective for lowering cholesterol as the statin drugs, despite their strong similarities. That may be because the dose wasn't high enough, or because the Cholestin capsules contained other substances or impurities that interfered with their lipid-lowering activity. Finally, more studies are needed to confirm that the findings from this trial are valid.

On the other hand, federal authorities closely regulate the purity of statin drugs. Years of research have demonstrated that these medications reduce the risk of heart disease. That can't be said about red yeast rice, which needs more study to show that it safely lowers the risk of heart attacks.

What else should I know about red yeast rice supplements?

No significant side effects were reported in the study mentioned above, though it only lasted a few months, so it's impossible to say whether long-term use of red yeast rice carries any risks. In rare cases, red yeast rice may cause serious food allergies that lead to anaphylactic shock.

If you're still confused—is red yeast rice a food, a dietary supplement, or a drug?—you're not alone. In recent years courts in the United States and the Food and Drug Administration have debated whether or not Cholestin is an unapproved drug.

Bottom line

If you have cholesterol problems that don't respond to diet and lifestyle changes, your physician can recommend treatment options that are well tested and proven safe. At this time, however, red yeast rice does not fit that description.

RIBOFLAVIN

Also known as Vitamin B$_2$

What is it?

Riboflavin is one of the B vitamins (see page 190). It's necessary for the formation of enzymes that help your body convert carbohydrates, fat, and protein in food into energy. Riboflavin is also needed for the other B vitamins to perform their functions. Deficiency of this nutrient is rare, but can cause mouth sores, skin problems, and even cataracts.

Grain manufacturers in the United States enrich bread, cereal, pasta, and rice with riboflavin and several other B vitamins that are lost during processing. Some other food sources of riboflavin include liver, milk, cheese, eggs, leafy green vegetables, whole grains, and brewer's yeast. The daily requirement of riboflavin is less than 2 milligrams for healthy adults, but riboflavin supplements (usually sold in pill form) often contain many times that amount. Furthermore, most multivitamins provide a day's worth of this nutrient.

Why do some people take riboflavin supplements?

Some migraine sufferers seek relief with these supplements. Riboflavin has also been recommended by some sources as a way to prevent or treat cataracts. Along with the other B vitamins, riboflavin is also included in "all-natural" arthritis preparations, too.

Do they work?

There is only a limited amount of research on the use of riboflavin to relieve migraines. In 1998, Belgian researchers reported that patients tormented by these crippling headaches experienced a 50 percent drop in attacks when they started taking 400 milligrams of riboflavin each day. However, this study involved a small number of patients; it's impossible to draw conclusions about the benefits and safety of riboflavin in treating migraines until further studies are performed. It's worth noting, however, that in this trial it took up to three or four months before the riboflavin supplements had any effect. Furthermore, when attacks did strike, riboflavin didn't appear to diminish their intensity or duration.

One potential effect of riboflavin deficiency is the formation of cataracts, which seems to have produced the theory that riboflavin supplements can prevent or treat this eye disease. Although Australian researchers found that people who eat foods rich in riboflavin have about half the risk of developing cataracts as people whose diets are low in riboflavin, it could be that riboflavin-rich foods provide some other source of nutrient for the eyes. Lacking formal trials, in which people who use riboflavin supplements are compared with nonusers, it's not possible to say whether megadoses of this nutrient prevent cataracts or restore sight.

Likewise, people with rheumatoid arthritis also tend to have low levels of riboflavin and other vitamins, but there's no solid evidence that vitamin supplements ease joint pain.

What else should I know about riboflavin supplements?

While riboflavin doesn't appear to cause significant side effects, more study is needed to determine whether megadoses are toxic.

Bottom line

Although it's an important nutrient, little is known about the use of riboflavin in supplement form to prevent or treat specific conditions. If you suffer from recurrent headaches or vision problems, see a physician.

ROYAL JELLY

What is it?

A cynic might call it bug spit. Technically, royal jelly is a milky fluid secreted by the salivary glands of worker bees. All baby bees, or grubs, feed on royal jelly, but only those destined to become queens are allowed to eat this prized substance for a lifetime. Royal jelly is about two-thirds water; the rest is made up of protein, sugars, and fat, with modest amounts of vitamins and minerals. Royal jelly is often blended with honey, as well as with ginseng and other herbs. Supplements are available in the form of capsules, liquid extract, and powder, as well as skin creams and lotions.

Why do some people take royal jelly supplements?

Queen bees grow to be twice the size of worker bees. They live much longer, too. These facts of nature have given rise to the belief that royal jelly is a superhealth tonic, providing youthful energy, promoting growth, and counteracting the effects of aging. Many other claims have been made about royal jelly over the years, including that it lowers cholesterol, strengthens the immune system, and clears up skin problems.

Do they work?

Yes, if you're a queen bee. But believing that the rest of us nonbees can benefit from royal jelly requires a huge leap of faith. No reliable research supports the suggestion that consuming these supplements will give you more energy or make you live longer. In fact, there's very little published research about the use of royal jelly by humans for any condition. The treatment of high cholesterol is one exception. A number of studies conducted in Europe and the former Soviet Union suggest that royal jelly may reduce levels of unhealthy blood fats. However, most of the studies involved small groups of patients, lasted a month or less, or had other design flaws that make their findings hard to trust.

All other uses of oral royal jelly supplements are based on anecdote, legend, or sketchy science. Likewise, claims that skin care products that contain royal jelly will clear up problems such as eczema and psoriasis are unproven. In fact, consuming royal jelly can lead to skin rashes and other problems (see below).

What else should I know about royal jelly supplements?

Anyone who is allergic to bees should avoid royal jelly or any other bee-related product. The medical literature is filled with reports of people who had bad reactions after using oral or topical royal jelly, including asthma attacks, hives, stomach pain, bloody diarrhea, chest pains, and facial swelling.

Bottom line

Don't rely on unproven therapies such as royal jelly to treat a serious condition such as elevated cholesterol. Talk to your physician about lifestyle changes and medications that have been proven to improve blood-fat profiles.

SAINT-JOHN'S-WORT

Scientific name: *Hypericum perforatum*

What is it?

Despite its rarified status in the world of medicinal herbs, Saint-John's-wort is a rather common plant. It grows all over the world, and to some gardeners the yellow-flowered perennial is nothing more than a weed. However, extract of the *Hypericum perforatum* has been prescribed to ease human suffering since the days of the ancient Greeks, who believed that it helped cure demonic possession. Today, Saint-John's-wort is one of the most widely used herbal therapies in Europe and the United States. In this country, it's usually sold in the form of capsules, liquid extract, or tea.

Why do some people take Saint-John's-wort supplements?

Although herbalists consider it a remedy for a variety of ailments, Saint-John's-wort is primarily used today to relieve depression.

Do they work?

A modest amount of clinical study suggests that a person with mild to moderate depression who takes Saint-John's-wort will feel somewhat better than if they take nothing at all. That was the conclusion reached by two separate groups of scientists who reviewed all the major studies conducted on the use of this herb for treating depression. Both groups determined that *Hypericum* extract consistently worked better than empty placebo pills.

However, a study published in the *Journal of the American Medical Association* found that Saint-John's-wort was *not* effective in the treatment of major depression. Furthermore, while this herb may be capable of favorably altering mood in less-severe cases of depression, much about it remains unclear. For starters, no one is sure how it works, nor has the specific active ingredient in Saint-John's-wort been identified with certainty. More important, little is known about how Saint-John's-wort stacks up against the most widely used antidepressant drugs. *Hypericum* extract has been found effective when compared with older medications that are rarely prescribed today, due to their severe side effects. But scientists are still trying to determine whether a depressed person benefits as much from taking Saint-John's-wort as from using one of the newer antidepressants, such as Prozac or Zoloft. A single small study suggests that may be true, but a large-scale trial—sponsored by the National Institutes of Health—involving more than three hundred people with moderately severe depression should shed more light on the therapeutic value of Saint-John's-wort.

What else should I know about Saint-John's-wort supplements?

Although many studies suggest that it causes fewer side effects than standard antidepressant drugs, Saint-John's-wort is by no means an entirely benign herb. To begin with, some side effects have been reported in users. They include nausea, fatigue, and a condition called photosensitivity, which makes the skin break out in a rash after even brief exposure to the sun. Saint-John's-wort can also interfere with the actions of a long list of medications, including drugs used to fight HIV infection, thin blood, prevent transplant rejections, and—ironically—treat depression. What's more, some reports suggest that Saint-John's-wort may also alter the effects of chemotherapy, birth control pills, and drugs used to prevent seizures and treat asthma and heart failure.

Evidence from some studies also raises the possibility that Saint-John's-wort may have effects similar to a class of antidepressants known as MAO inhibitors. Patients who use MAO inhibitors are given strict orders to avoid certain foods and beverages, such as cheese and red wine, because when combined with these drugs they can cause dangerously high blood pressure. In theory, Saint-John's-wort may be unsafe to consume in combination with red wine and cheese, too. Some evidence suggests that this herb may also interfere with the body's ability to absorb iron.

Bottom line

Some preliminary studies suggest that Saint-John's-wort is effective in relieving the symptoms of mild depression, but other evidence suggests that it may have no value. What's more, too little is known about how this herb works, whether it's safe to use, and whether it's as effective as carefully tested antidepressant drugs.

In 1998 the *Los Angeles Times* commissioned a lab analysis of various brands of Saint-John's-wort to determine whether they contained the level of active ingredient stated on the label; seven out of ten brands flunked.

SAMe

Scientific name: S-adenosyl-methionine

What is it?

SAMe (pronounced "sammy") is a naturally occurring molecule that acts as an intermediary in many important biochemical reactions in the human body. A typical diet provides an insignificant amount of SAMe, so your body makes its own supply. As a dietary supplement, SAMe is sold in tablet form.

Why do some people take SAMe?

In some European countries, SAMe is prescribed as a drug to treat depression. The publication of several books, including *Stop Depression Now*, heightened interest in SAMe's mood-enhancing capabilities in this country. SAMe is also said to relieve the pain of arthritis and fibromyalgia (a condition that causes sore joints and fatigue) and repair damaged livers.

Does it work?

SAMe quickly became one of the hottest-selling dietary supplements in the United States after its introduction on these shores in 1999. TV talk shows and magazine articles featured testimonials from people who said the pills had brightened their spirits and ended years of sore joints. But despite the hype, there are still many unresolved questions about this so-called natural blues buster and pain reliever.

SAMe's reputation as a mood lifter is based largely on a series of studies showing that the compound is more effective than sugar pills in treating depression. Viewed as a group, these studies also suggest that SAMe works about as well as a class of antidepressants known as tricyclics. Scientists have proposed that SAMe may make brain cells more fluid, allowing chemical messengers called neurotransmitters to move about more freely.

However, a closer look at the studies that have helped build SAMe's reputation reveals that they don't tell us much about the pills sold in this country. First, very small groups of patients were tested—far fewer than would be required to get a drug approved in the United States. Furthermore, most of these studies used a form of SAMe that's injected into the body. The SAMe packed in pills may not act the same as intravenous SAMe. Any medication that's taken orally must dissolve efficiently in the lower intestine to reach the bloodstream. There's reason to believe that some people may not absorb enough SAMe to have a therapeutic effect.

In other words, even if injected SAMe treats depression, one can't assume that oral SAMe will do the same. Unfortunately, there have only been a few small studies of oral SAMe in depressed people. SAMe pills need to be tested in larger groups of patients with depression to determine whether they're safe and effective. In particular, SAMe needs to be compared side by side with commonly prescribed antidepressants such as Prozac and other related drugs (known as selective serotonin reuptake inhibitors, or SSRIs) before we can understand its true value.

Even less is known about SAMe's ability to numb physical pain. Aside from a few small studies, there has been little research involving people with arthritis and fibromyalgia, two conditions said to respond well to SAMe. This supplement is also touted as beneficial for people with liver disease. But liver damage must be evaluated by a physician, who can prescribe an appropriate course of therapy.

What else should I know about SAMe?

Proponents say that SAMe acts faster than standard antidepressants and has virtually no side effects, though its safety hasn't been adequately studied. There have been anecdotal reports of SAMe users who developed the psychiatric disorder known as manic depression. SAMe is converted to a substance called homocysteine, which has been associated with an increased risk of cardiovascular disease. In theory, taking SAMe supplements could raise homocysteine levels.

Bottom line

SAMe pills have never been proven effective in the treatment of depression or pain in formal studies. Furthermore, there's no solid information about the short- and long-term safety of using SAMe.

SAW PALMETTO

Scientific name: *Serenoa repens*

What is it?

This small palmlike tree, which grows in Florida and other parts of the southeastern United States, yields berries that are used medicinally either fresh or dried. The latter form is used to make tea, but it's more commonly consumed in capsule form.

Why do some people take saw palmetto supplements?

To treat the symptoms of an enlarged prostate, also known as benign prostatic hypertrophy (BPH), which is common in men over forty. An enlarged prostate can inhibit the flow of urine, causing men to feel a frequent need to urinate, particularly at night and often with unsatisfying results. Some men with BPH end up retaining urine, which can lead to bladder infections.

Some women use saw palmetto in the belief that it will enlarge their breasts. The herb is occasionally found in preparations that allegedly increase sexual desire and potency.

Do they work?

Most studies of saw palmetto for the treatment of BPH have been on the small side, involving considerably fewer subjects than would be required for approval of a prescription drug in the United States. However, several reviews of the existing medical literature on this increasingly popular herb have determined that it probably does improve urinary flow in men with BPH, though the effect may be modest. Although saw palmetto should be studied further, there's some evidence that it treats the symptoms of an enlarged prostate about as well as standard drug therapy, with fewer side effects, such as erectile dysfunction.

Saw palmetto acts much like the drug finasteride (sold under the brand name Proscar), which shrinks an enlarged prostate by altering the way the hormone testosterone is processed in the body. Scientists are currently studying whether finasteride's influence on male hormones can help prevent prostate cancer. But it's too soon to say whether finasteride or saw palmetto has a role in cancer prevention.

One recent study found that men taking saw palmetto did not experience any changes in their libido or sexual potency, casting doubt on the herb's use in aphrodisiac preparations sold on the Internet and elsewhere. In fact, since saw palmetto may interfere with the production of male hormones, one might expect it to have the opposite effect, at least in theory. Likewise, there's no scientific proof that consuming this herb will increase breast size.

What else should I know about saw palmetto supplements?

Other than mild stomach upset, saw palmetto causes few known side effects, though some could emerge as the herb undergoes closer scientific scrutiny. Saw palmetto may interfere with the body's ability to absorb iron. Consuming saw palmetto may cause a slight change in a man's levels of prostate specific antigen (PSA), which is a protein produced by the prostate. When doctors screen for prostate cancer they measure PSA levels, which often change in men who have the disease. Since the presence of saw palmetto could alter the results of a PSA test, men who take the herb should tell their physicians.

Bottom line

Saw palmetto appears to shrink the prostate, relieving the symptoms of BPH. But since this herb acts a lot like a drug, a physician should monitor anyone who uses it. Don't self-treat BPH; its symptoms are similar to those of other, more serious conditions, including prostate cancer. All men should talk to their doctors about prostate cancer screening.

SELENIUM

What is it?

Selenium is a trace mineral found throughout the body. A potent antioxidant, it is thought to protect cells and arteries from damage by naturally occurring substances in the body called free radicals. Rich sources of selenium include Brazil nuts, whole grains, seafood, egg yolk, garlic, and brewer's yeast. The selenium content of grains and vegetables depends largely on where they're grown, since the mineral composition of soil varies by region. Likewise, livestock fed grains low in selenium will also have low levels of the mineral. Selenium capsules and tablets are widely available, and the mineral is found in multivitamins.

Why do some people take selenium supplements?

To prevent cancer. Selenium is also sometimes included in regimens of antioxidant supplements intended to battle cardiovascular disease.

Do they work?

Scientists have been studying the link between selenium and cancer since the late 1960s, and have turned up some intriguing evidence in recent years. According to a 1996 study reported in the *Journal of the American Medical Association*, people who took 200 micrograms of selenium a day had a 63 percent lower risk of prostate cancer than people who took inactive placebo pills. The selenium group also appeared to lower their risk for lung and colon cancer, too. (Interestingly, the study involved people with a history of skin cancer and was designed to determine whether selenium prevents the recurrence of that disease, which it did not.)

Another study, from China, suggests that selenium supplements (as well as vitamin E and beta carotene pills) may reduce the risk of dying from cancer. Based on the findings from these studies, scientists are trying to determine whether selenium supplements can help prevent a specific cancer—prostate cancer, which afflicts nearly 200,000 American men each year. (Vitamin E supplements are also being studied for the same purpose.) With the completion of this large study, which will involve over 32,000 men, doctors will be able to say with greater confidence whether or not selenium supplements have the potential to fight cancer.

As an antioxidant, selenium should be good for the heart, but whether taking high-dose supplements prevents heart disease remains an unanswered question. Selenium is sometimes recommended for other conditions, including rheumatoid arthritis, but the evidence is either contradictory or incomplete.

What else should I know about selenium supplements?

At very high doses, selenium can cause loss of hair and nails, skin damage, and neurological problems.

Bottom line

Some preliminary research suggests that selenium supplements may help prevent cancer. However, until this antioxidant mineral has been studied more closely, it's too soon to recommend selenium supplements for that purpose.

SHARK CARTILAGE

What is it?

The skeletons of sharks caught in the Pacific Ocean are ground up and sold in several forms, including powders and capsules.

Why do some people take shark cartilage supplements?

Although some use these supplements to treat arthritis, shark cartilage is best known as a treatment for cancer, and a highly controversial one at that. Thanks in large part to a 1992 book promoting the supplements, titled *Sharks Don't Get Cancer*, about fifty thousand Americans suffering from various forms of the disease use shark cartilage supplements each year.

Do they work?

Surprise—sharks *do* get cancer, as researchers at George Washington University have shown. The unproven and questionable theory that shark cartilage supplements fight the disease dates back to the early 1980s. Research in animals found that shark cartilage appeared to contain substances that slowed down angiogenesis, or the growth of blood vessels, around tumors. In theory, cutting off the blood supply to a tumor should cause it to stop growing.

However, that theory hasn't held up when shark cartilage was studied under the kinds of conditions used to test prescription drugs. Even if something in the ground-up shark skeleton can stop the growth of blood vessels, most researchers agree that there's little chance that the body would absorb enough of it to have any therapeutic effect. There has only been a handful of studies in which shark cartilage was formally tested in animals and humans for the treatment of cancer. So far, the supplements appear to be worthless.

If you need any further reason to be skeptical, take note that the Federal Trade Commission has issued stiff fines to several companies that sell shark cartilage supplements for making unsubstantiated claims that their products prevented and cured cancer.

There is no scientific evidence that shark cartilage supplements treat the symptoms of arthritis, either.

What else should I know about shark cartilage supplements?

People who use these supplements sometimes complain of upset stomach, weakness, dizziness, and a foul taste in the mouth.

Shark cartilage supplements don't live up to their hype, but there is new hope for cancer patients. Many new drugs are being developed, some of which inhibit angiogenesis and other processes that cause cancer to spread. Clinical trials involving these new drugs are usually available for patients when standard therapies prove ineffective.

Bottom line

If you're looking for new options in cancer treatment, don't go to your local vitamin store. Talk to your physician about clinical trials, which test new drugs in carefully controlled settings.

SIBERIAN GINSENG

Scientific name: *Eleutherococcus senticosus*
Also known as eleuthero and Russian ginseng

What is it?

Herbalists consider the name a misnomer, since Siberian ginseng does not belong to the same species as Asian ginseng or American ginseng, though it is classified in the same plant family. This deciduous shrub grows throughout China, Japan, Korea, and Russia. The root of the *Eleutherococcus senticosus* is pulverized and processed as an extract that is sold in many forms, including capsules, drops, powders, teas, and soft drinks.

Why do some people take Siberian ginseng supplements?

Like other varieties of ginseng, this herb is thought of as an all-natural source of energy and strength, one that's particularly beneficial for stressful times. Russian scientists who first proposed Siberian ginseng as a cheaper alternative to Asian and American ginseng believed that it acts as an equally strong adaptogen, which is a nonmedical term for any substance that bolsters physical and mental well-being.

Do they work?

Siberian ginseng's reputation as an all-around performance booster can be traced to studies performed on Russian athletes in the 1960s and 1970s. However, American scientists have criticized the quality of this research as being biased in a way guaranteed to yield positive results. A more recent study of Siberian ginseng's effect on exercise performance found no benefit. Researchers gave 3.4 milligrams of *Eleutherococcus senticosus* liquid extract to twenty distance runners every day for six weeks. The athletes' level of conditioning didn't change, suggesting that the Siberian ginseng had no effect. It's possible that the runners had already reached peak levels of strength and endurance, and that less-fit people might benefit from Siberian ginseng. But until more studies are conducted, the value of this herb as a botanical pick-me-up can't be confirmed.

Most doctors in the West don't believe in the existence of adaptogens, since the concept is based on a theory that's not supported by scientific evidence. Some researchers have suggested that Siberian ginseng may have a direct effect on the human immune system, though whether that's true—and whether the effect would even be beneficial—isn't clear.

What else should I know about Siberian ginseng supplements?

There are few known side effects associated with this herb, although long-term studies of its use have not been performed. There are reports in the medical literature that Siberian ginseng may interfere with the accuracy of a blood test used to monitor levels of the drug digoxin, which is often prescribed to patients suffering from heart failure. The presence of this herb may also affect the activity of drugs intended to thin blood, control heart rate, and treat diabetes.

Bottom line

Siberian ginseng and its herbal cousin, *Panax ginseng*, have enjoyed huge popularity among American consumers in recent years. But the widespread belief that they boost human performance—whether on a playing field or in a boardroom—isn't backed up by a solid body of scientific evidence.

SOY AND SOY ISOFLAVONES

What are they?

Soybeans were first grown in northern China, perhaps as long as four thousand years ago. This legume is rich in protein, which is why it's so popular among vegetarians (meat being a main source of protein in the American diet). Soybeans are used to make a head-spinning array of food products—everything from soy sauce to tofu hot dogs. Along with all that protein, soy also contains compounds known as isoflavones (pronounced "ice-oh-FLAY-voanz") that act as antioxidants. Some isoflavones are chemically similar to the hormone estrogen.

Soy dietary supplements are sold in many forms, including capsules, tablets, powdered beverages, and energy bars. Some products are designed to contain high doses of isoflavones.

Why do some people take soy supplements?

To lower cholesterol and reduce the risk of various cancers. Soy is also sometimes recommended to build stronger bones and ease post-menopausal symptoms, such as hot flashes.

Do they work?

There are good reasons to add soy foods to your diet. However, recommending dietary supplements that contain soy is a little trickier, as you'll see.

Heart disease

An analysis of several studies found that eating 47 grams of soy protein each day instead of animal protein lowered total cholesterol by 9 percent and LDL ("bad") cholesterol by nearly 13 percent. Granted, that's a lot of soy. You need to eat about a block of tofu each day to consume the equivalent of 47 grams of soy protein. However, other studies show that adding even a small serving of soy to the daily diet can result in a modest drop in total cholesterol. And if you're at risk for heart disease, every little bit may help. According to one formula, for every 1 percent you lower your total cholesterol, your risk for heart disease drops by 2 percent. Furthermore, lowering the ratio of LDL ("bad") cholesterol to HDL ("good") cholesterol also reduces the risk for heart disease.

Cancer

In Japan, death rates from breast and prostate cancers are three or four times lower than in the United States. Some scientists believe that the Japanese gain cancer protection from the soy in their diets. Although not proven, soy may decrease the risk of breast cancer because it contains plant estrogens (known as phytoestrogens). Naturally occurring estrogen in women can act on cell receptors to promote the growth of breast cancer and some other cancers. According to one theory, phytoestrogens—which are weaker hormones—may protect breast tissue by competing with human estrogen for those same cell receptors. In men, phytoestrogens may inhibit the growth of prostate cancer, though whether soy has a role in preventing this disease isn't known.

In fact, it's fair to say that soy's role in cancer prevention is still somewhat mysterious, if it has a beneficial role at all. After all, the low cancer rates in Japan may have nothing to do with soy. To complicate matters further, a 1999 study found that healthy women who took a soy supplement for two weeks (60 grams daily) showed evidence of estrogenic activity in their breasts. Scientists believe that high doses of the hormone estrogen increase the risk of uterine cancers, and possibly breast cancer, so it's logical to assume that high doses of plant estrogens might do the same. But how does that possibility square with the theory that moderate doses of soy *protect* against breast cancer? No one is sure, but some studies suggest that age, dose, or the type of phytoestrogen may be important factors. It could be that phytoestrogens act differently in the young than they do in older people.

Perhaps the best interpretation of this apparently contradictory information is that more study is needed to understand the relationship between soy and cancer.

Bone health and postmenopausal symptoms

Asian women have lower rates of bone fractures than women in the West. There has been only limited clinical research on the influence of soy on human bones, and so far the evidence is ambiguous. One study showed that a large daily dose (40 grams of soy protein) significantly increased bone density in middle-aged and elderly women after six months. However, another study of nearly 500 postmenopausal women, published in the *Journal of the American Medical Association,* found that a supplement containing a soy derivative (known as ipriflavone) does not prevent bone loss. If soy fights osteoporosis, it may be due to its high levels of phytoestrogens. It's known, after all, that postmenopausal women who use prescription estrogen-replacement therapy (ERT) develop stronger bones and have few problems with hot flashes and vaginal dryness. In theory, the phytoestrogens in soy and other plant foods should act like ERT.

Here's one potential catch: It's known that ERT also increases the risk of uterine cancer and may increase the risk of breast cancer. However, women who have an intact uterus who are treated with prescription hormones are also given progesterone, which reduces the risk of uterine cancer (as well as ovarian cancer). Theoretically, a woman who consumes large amounts of phytoestrogens, from soy or any other source, might increase her risk for these diseases—but will lack the protective effects of progesterone.

American women are four times more likely than Chinese women to experience hot flashes after reaching menopause. As in Japan, soy foods are a staple of the Chinese diet. But, again, it's not clear that soy is the solution. Trials designed to test the cooling powers of soy foods have shown only modest benefits, if any at all, for women plagued by hot flashes. Furthermore, any benefits soy might have in fighting hot flashes have to be balanced against the concern that some estrogens may increase cancer risk.

There's not enough information to draw conclusions about soy's usefulness in treating other health problems, such as vaginal dryness, experienced by postmenopausal women.

Deciding which soy foods or supplements to eat for good health can be confusing. Soy powdered drink mixes have been used in many research trials and may be a convenient alternative for people who won't eat tofu or other soy foods. However, soy pills haven't been well studied.

Scientists are still trying to sort out whether it's the protein, isoflavones, or some other component of soy—or all of them working together—that may provide health benefits. The labels of some dietary supplements don't specify the isoflavone content, while others make a point of boasting that they're loaded with these phytoestrogens. To add to the confusion, the isoflavone levels in the many different soy foods vary greatly. For instance, soy yogurt is about twice as high in isoflavones by weight as a soy burger.

What else should I know about soy supplements?

Humans have been eating soy for millennia. There has been little reason to question its safety until recently, though this research needs to be viewed in proper perspective. Theoretically, very high doses of soy phytoestrogens could be harmful, although our understanding of how these compounds work is still not clear. Keep this point in mind, however: most concerns about this plant food are focused on soy derivatives sold in supplements. There's little reason to believe there's any danger in eating moderate amounts of soy as part of a healthy, balanced diet.

Researchers in Hawaii found that Japanese-American men who ate a lot of tofu in middle age appeared to develop symptoms of dementia earlier in life than men who avoided soybean curd. However, this much-hyped study only showed an association between eating soy foods and developing cognitive problems. It does not represent proof that consuming tofu causes such an effect, which would require much more research.

Bottom line

Studies suggest that adding soy foods to your diet may reduce the risk of cardiovascular disease, though their role in cancer prevention isn't well understood. Taking supplements that contain phytoestrogens to relieve postmenopausal symptoms is inadvisable, since they could theoretically carry significant health risks. Furthermore, pills and powders that contain soy protein or compounds extracted from soybeans may be missing important components found in soy foods. To be on the safe side, talk to your physician about the proper role for soy in your diet, and be sure to discuss all the steps you can take to prevent heart disease and cancer. Women who are bothered by symptoms related to menopause should seek medical advice about all available treatment options.

SPIRULINA

Scientific names: *Spirulina maxima, S. platensis*, and others
Also known as blue-green algae

What is it?

Spirulina is a type of blue-green algae that forms on the surface of ponds and lakes all over the world (sometimes known as slime or pond scum). Historically, some cultures have harvested spirulina to be dried and eaten. Since the late 1970s, health food stores in this country have sold spirulina and other forms of blue-green algae as pills and powders, the latter for sprinkling on foods or dissolving in beverages.

Why do some people take spirulina supplements?

Spirulina proponents claim that it's a kind of superfood, packed with high doses of protein, vitamins, minerals, and other vital nutrients. They also insist that spirulina has an astonishing range of healthful properties, able to lower the risk of heart disease, cancer, and liver disease, while also fighting allergies and strengthening the immune system. Spirulina and blue-green algae are also said to aid in weight loss.

Do they work?

There's little science to support all the hype over spirulina. Virtually all health claims you're likely to hear or read about these green pills and powders are based on untested theories, anecdotal reports, or a limited amount of test-tube and animal research. For example, a few studies involving lab rats are the basis for claims that spirulina will improve cholesterol levels. Spirulina's reputation as a diet aid hinges on the theory that a substance in spirulina suppresses appetite. But this theory has never been proven, and there are no reliable studies to show that spirulina speeds weight loss.

If you're thinking about taking spirulina strictly for its highly touted nutrient content, consider a few facts first. As a source of protein, spirulina is very expensive compared to lean meats or low-fat dairy products. There's also some evidence that nutrients in spirulina aren't what they appear to be. For example, companies often describe spirulina as "nature's richest source of vitamin B_{12}." Yet, one analysis determined that 80 percent of the "vitamin B_{12}" in several samples of spirulina turned out to be substances that are similar to this important vitamin, but have little or no known nutritional value to humans.

A study of tobacco chewers that was performed in India found that spirulina may be able to eliminate lesions, or sores, that can lead to oral cancer. However, in many cases the lesions eventually returned, and a larger study would be necessary to understand whether spirulina prevents any type of cancer.

What else should I know about spirulina supplements?

Given the lack of research on spirulina and blue-green algae in humans, it's impossible to say whether these products are safe to use. The purity of some spirulina products has been questioned; one popular source, a lake in Oregon, turned out to be polluted with bird droppings in 1996. Liver-damaging toxins were detected in one analysis of spirulina tablets sold in health food stores.

About the kindest term you'll hear used to describe the taste of spirulina is "earthy."

Bottom line

Don't believe the hype about these exotic-sounding products. Spirulina and blue-green algae have no proven role in improving human health.

THIAMIN

Also known as thiamine and vitamin B_1

What is it?

Thiamin is one of the B vitamins (see page 190). It has a number of essential roles in the human body. One is to help break down carbohydrates in food and use them as energy. Your body doesn't store large amounts of thiamin, so you need to replenish your supply every day. Thiamin deficiency can lead to the neurological disease known as beriberi, which is practically unknown in the United States, largely because cereals, breads, pasta, and rice are enriched with the nutrient. What's more, thiamin occurs naturally in pork, organ meats, beans, peas, nuts, eggs, and other foods. Thiamin pills are available, and the nutrient is also found in multivitamins.

Why do some people take thiamin supplements?

Long-term, heavy drinking can cause thiamin deficiency, so physicians often prescribe these supplements to alcoholics. Like other B vitamins, thiamin is often included in stress-formula dietary supplements, which allegedly combat mental tension. Athletes have been known to take thiamin supplements, believing that high doses of the nutrient improve endurance.

Do they work?

It's not yet clear whether there's any reason to use these supplements for any purpose other than treating thiamin deficiency. However, some researchers believe thiamin supplements may improve cognitive function in both healthy and diseased people. So far, their work has yielded some interesting—if preliminary—results. For example, Welsh researchers found that healthy young women improved their mental sharpness after taking a daily 50-milligram supplement of thiamin for two months. This and the few other studies of thiamin as food for the brain need to be confirmed by more research. Likewise, there's not much evidence to support using thiamin supplements if you want to exercise longer or harder. Endurance athletes do require more thiamin than nonathletes, but the extra nutrition is easily obtained through a well-balanced diet.

What else should I know about thiamin supplements?

Thiamin appears to be a safe vitamin, although there have been reports of severe side effects when it's consumed in massive doses. Most multivitamins contain the daily requirement for thiamin.

Bottom line

Thiamin may be a critical nutrient, but a balanced diet provides adequate levels for most people.

Some outdoorsy types take thiamin supplements in the unproven belief that high levels of the vitamin—which is partially excreted through the skin—help ward off mosquitoes.

VALERIAN

Scientific name: *Valeriana officinalis*

What is it?

This tall perennial plant with pink flowers grows in temperate climates in many parts of the world. Valerian is the common name for a genus that includes various species, but *Valeriana officinalis* is the one most frequently used medicinally. The underground stems and roots are dried and processed, usually as capsules, liquid extract, or tea.

Why do some people take valerian supplements?

To get a better night's sleep. According to a survey by the National Sleep Foundation, nearly two-thirds of American adults have trouble getting to sleep at least a few nights per week. About one person in twelve suffers from chronic insomnia.

Do they work?

In several controlled studies, many people plagued by troubled sleep reported that they dozed off faster and rested more soundly on nights when they took valerian supplements before going to bed. For example, in one trial, 54 percent of study subjects who were characterized as "habitually poor or irregular sleepers" said they improved the quality of their sleep after taking valerian.

But while these studies are interesting, a few caveats are worth noting. First, one of them was rather modest in size, involving fewer than thirty people. Furthermore, some studies relied on self reports—that is, the subjects were asked to evaluate their own sleep on nights when they were taking valerian versus nights when they were given empty placebo pills. Because valerian has a distinct odor (many would say offensive), it's possible that some of the subjects knew when they were popping the herb, which might bias their feelings about how they slept.

Using a different approach, one of these research teams gave valerian to another group of people who complained of poor sleep, only this time special equipment was used to estimate how long it took them to drift off. The team determined that taking valerian reduced the amount of time it took to fall asleep from about sixteen minutes to nine minutes. Again, however, this study involved just a handful of subjects. Valerian may work as a mild sedative, but it will take large, well-designed trials to confirm that theory once and for all.

What else should I know about valerian supplements?

Few side effects have been reported among people who use this herb, though headaches, heart palpitations, and—ironically—insomnia can occur. Because valerian may make you sleepy, don't use it if you have to drive or do any other task that requires alertness. It's probably unwise to consume alcohol or use any other sedative with valerian. If your doctor has prescribed iron supplements to treat a deficiency in the mineral, avoid valerian.

Valerian may also pose problems when you stop using it. The *New England Journal of Medicine* reported the case of a patient who quit taking the herb and experienced serious withdrawal symptoms, including elevated blood pressure and heart rate, similar to those felt by patients who go off standard antianxiety medications.

Finally, there's that odor. This scent of valerian has been compared to dirty sweat socks, which helps explain one of this plant's nicknames: stinkweed.

Bottom line

Until more research is conducted to understand how valerian works, this herb should be avoided. There's good reason to believe that valerian may act like antianxiety medications, which can have serious side effects.

VANADYL SULFATE

Also known as vanadium

What is it?

First, you need to know about vanadium, which is a nonessential trace mineral. In other words, it has some of the qualities of other trace minerals, but has not been proven necessary for human health. Vanadium's role in the body isn't well understood, but animal studies suggest that it enhances the effect of insulin. Specifically, vanadium appears to help cells use carbohydrates as energy. Vanadium is usually sold in pill form as vanadyl sulfate.

Why do some people take vanadyl sulfate supplements?

Vanadyl sulfate is popular with bodybuilders, many of whom believe the supplements boost muscle size in a way similar to anabolic steroids. Some proponents of alternative medicine recommend vanadyl sulfate to diabetics, claiming that it's a safe and proven substitute for insulin.

Do they work?

There is no solid scientific evidence that taking vanadyl sulfate builds bigger muscles in humans. The theory comes from lab and animal studies, which suggested that the mineral compound may increase lean tissue. In one study designed to examine whether vanadyl sulfate makes muscle in humans, scientists compared two groups of men and women involved in strength training for twelve weeks. One group took vanadyl sulfate supplements; the other didn't. At the end of the study, scientists detected no difference between the two groups in body composition.

Although some small studies suggest that vanadyl sulfate may help control blood sugar levels, it's unwise for anyone with diabetes to self-treat this very serious condition. That's especially true with vanadyl sulfate, since some research shows that it may cause serious side effects (see next section).

What else should I know about vanadyl sulfate supplements?

Short-term studies have found vanadyl sulfate to be reasonably safe, causing only minor stomach problems. However, some evidence suggests that long-term use could result in liver or kidney damage.

Bottom line

Although some preliminary studies suggest that vanadyl sulfate may improve glucose utilization in patients with diabetes, there's not enough scientific evidence to recommend these supplements for this or any other purpose.

VITAMIN A

What is it?

Vitamin A is actually a group of compounds, known collectively as the retinoids. You might call it the vision vitamin, since vitamin A is critical for healthy eyes, particularly for seeing in dim light. But this vitamin, the first discovered, plays many other vital roles in the human body. Without vitamin A your skin would turn dry and hard, as would the lining of the internal organs, leaving you vulnerable to infections. Vitamin A, particularly in the form of retinoic acid, is necessary for healthy cells, making them less likely to grow uncontrollably and form tumors.

Vitamin A deficiency is a huge problem in the developing world, each year causing millions of cases of childhood blindness and other diseases. In industrialized countries, chronic lack of vitamin A is far less common, but it does occur and can lead to night blindness, total blindness, and a long list of other conditions.

We get about half of our vitamin A from animal foods and the other half from plant foods (in the form of carotenoids, which the body converts to vitamin A). Dairies in the United States fortify milk with this important vitamin, too. Vitamin A is usually the first ingredient listed on a bottle of multivitamins and you can also buy individual vitamin A pills.

Why do some people use vitamin A supplements?

Supplement sellers often promote vitamin A as critical for healthy skin and strong eyes. In particular, it's often used in preparations said to cure night blindness and improve overall vision. Vitamin A is often included in so-called immune-booster supplements, whose ads hint that high doses of the nutrient will prevent cancer.

Do they work?

For the average person, there's probably little benefit to taking commercially available vitamin A supplements. The only reason they would improve the appearance of your skin or your vision would be if you suffer from a vitamin A deficiency, which is rare—and would require the attention of a physician, anyway.

Vitamin A is being studied for its potential role in preventing cancer, particularly skin cancer. But the research so far has yielded inconclusive results (and has typically involved derivatives of vitamin A you're not apt to find at your local health food store). Of greater concern, in some studies supplements of vitamin A and beta carotene (which the body converts to vitamin A) appeared to be dangerous, apparently increasing the risk of lung cancer in smokers.

What else should I know about vitamin A supplements?

Taking a lot of vitamin A over an extended period can lead to a laundry list of maladies, ranging from the merely unpleasant (such as dry skin) to the very serious (such as liver disease). Women who are planning to become pregnant shouldn't take high doses of vitamin A, since it has been linked to birth defects.

A prescription drug derivative of vitamin A, retinoic acid, is available for the treatment of acne.

Bottom line

Unless your physician determines that you're deficient in vitamin A, there's little reason to take these supplements—which, at high doses, could make you very sick.

VITAMIN B COMPLEX

See separate entries for thiamin, riboflavin, vitamin B$_6$, niacin, pantothenic acid, biotin, folic acid, and vitamin B$_{12}$.

What is it?

Vitamin B complex is the name for a group of vitamins that includes thiamin (also known as vitamin B$_1$), riboflavin (vitamin B$_2$), pyridoxine (usually known as vitamin B$_6$), niacin, pantothenic acid, biotin, folic acid, and cyanocobalamin (known as vitamin B$_{12}$). Each vitamin has a unique job, but generally speaking the B complex helps to form cells and convert the food you eat into energy. Your body can't store large amounts of the B vitamins, so you need a fresh dose every day. Fortunately, they're present in many foods, including breads and other grain products, which by law must be enriched with these vitamins in the United States. Vitamin B deficiency is rare in this country.

Vitamin B complex supplements—which contain varying degrees of all the B vitamins—are widely available. You can also purchase pills packed with the individual B vitamins.

Why do some people take vitamin B complex supplements?

Supplement sellers claim these combination pills relieve stress, boost mood, and fight fatigue, while restoring vitamins allegedly depleted by an "active lifestyle."

Do they work?

Physicians prescribe vitamin B complex to patients diagnosed with conditions that cause vitamin B deficiency, including alcoholism. Some study suggests that people suffering from chronic fatigue have reduced levels of B vitamins. However, there's no solid proof that popping a vitamin B complex supplement can erase everyday tension and mental weariness. Furthermore, B vitamins are plentiful in a balanced diet, so there's no reason to think that people with "active lifestyles" need extra-high doses.

On the other hand, several of the individual B vitamins may be useful for specific conditions. For example, folic acid, vitamin B$_6$, and vitamin B$_{12}$ lower levels of homocysteine, a substance found in the blood that may increase the risk for cardiovascular disease. Ongoing research will attempt to determine whether consuming these vitamins in the form of dietary supplements can protect against heart attacks.

What else should I know about vitamin B complex supplements?

Vitamin B is generally safe, as long as you stick to the recommended daily allowances. Still, it's always a good idea to read bottle labels to know how much of each individual vitamin you're getting, since there's no standard formulation for vitamin B complex supplements.

If you're chronically stressed out, find a relaxation technique—such as meditation, prayer, deep breathing, or fly-fishing—that works for you, and stick with it. Fatigue usually responds well to a very old remedy—eight hours of shut-eye every night. If you're getting plenty of sleep but still lack energy, see your physician.

Bottom line

Several of the B vitamins may prove useful in preventing cardiovascular disease by controlling homocysteine levels, though you should talk to a medical doctor before taking any supplement for that purpose. While you're at it, be sure to ask your doctor about controlling other well-established risk factors for heart disease, such as elevated cholesterol and blood pressure.

VITAMIN B$_6$

Also known as pyridoxine

What is it?

Vitamin B$_6$ is actually a collection of several related substances that together play a wide variety of roles in the human body. Vitamin B$_6$ is critical for metabolizing food into energy and converting the amino acid tryptophan into niacin (see page 144). It's also necessary for producing muscle and other tissue, as well as hormones and other chemicals required for a healthy nervous system (including serotonin, which appears to help regulate mood). Along with folate (see page 94), another B vitamin, B$_6$ lowers blood levels of homocysteine, an amino acid that may increase the risk of heart disease.

Vitamin B$_6$ deficiency is uncommon. Meats, whole grains, soybeans, peanuts, wheat germ, and brewer's yeast are all rich in this nutrient. Vitamin B$_6$ supplements are widely available; the vitamin is also included in multivitamins and B complex supplements.

Why do some people take vitamin B$_6$ supplements?

Given the long list of functions vitamin B$_6$ plays in the body, it's no surprise that supplements containing the substance are used or studied for the prevention and treatment of many different conditions. A few of the more common include asthma, carpal tunnel syndrome, depression and anxiety, heart disease, kidney stones, and premenstrual syndrome. Vitamin B$_6$ supplements are also used to strengthen the immune system, your body's infection fighter.

Do they work?

The most intense scientific interest in vitamin B$_6$ in recent years has concerned its role in preventing cardiovascular disease. Several studies published in the 1990s determined that people with high blood levels of the amino acid homocysteine had an increased risk for heart disease. Eating foods that contain vitamin B$_6$, as well as folic acid and vitamin B$_{12}$, can lower homocysteine levels.

A 1998 study offers some evidence (though hardly conclusive) that vitamin B$_6$ is good for the cardiovascular system. Harvard researchers amassed nutritional data on over eighty thousand female nurses and found that women who took supplements containing vitamin B$_6$ cut their risk of having a heart attack by one-third. Taking supplemental vitamin B$_6$ *and* folate offered even more protection.

Other ongoing trials are probing the link between cardiovascular health and homocysteine levels—specifically, whether lowering homocysteine with vitamin B$_6$ (as well as vitamin B$_{12}$ and folate) prevents heart attacks and strokes. As for the many other conditions for which vitamin B$_6$ has been studied, there is some interesting evidence, but no sure things. Furthermore, the idea of taking high doses of vitamin B$_6$ for long periods worries many doctors, and with good reason (see next item).

What else should I know about vitamin B$_6$ supplements?

Vitamin B$_6$ can be toxic at high doses, causing loss of muscle coordination and nerve damage.

Bottom line

More study is needed to determine whether lowering high homocysteine levels—whether with vitamin B$_6$ supplements or any other means—prevents heart attacks and strokes—and whether supplements of vitamin B$_6$ or other nutrients cause such a decrease. A blood test can determine homocysteine levels; ask your doctor if you're an appropriate candidate for this test. (See the separate entry for folic acid, page 94, to learn more about homocysteine and dietary supplements.)

VITAMIN B$_{12}$

Also known as cobalamin and cyanocobalamin

What is it?

The most recently discovered of the B vitamins, this essential nutrient is involved in the formation of red blood cells, the production of DNA, and the manufacture of myelin sheaths that protect nerves. Your body also needs vitamin B$_{12}$ to use another B vitamin, folate (see page 94), and to metabolize food.

Vitamin B$_{12}$ deficiency is often caused by a condition called pernicious anemia, which can lead to weakness and tingling in the extremities, among other symptoms. Also, some vegans—whose diets exclude animal products—can develop vitamin B$_{12}$ deficiency. Rich dietary sources include meats, fish, and dairy products. As a dietary supplement, vitamin B$_{12}$ is sold in capsule form and is included in most multivitamins. Injections are available in doctor's offices.

Why do some people take vitamin B$_{12}$ supplements?

Doctors treat pernicious anemia with injections of vitamin B$_{12}$. Some sufferers of chronic fatigue syndrome supplement their diets with high doses of this vitamin. It used to be fashionable for rock stars and other celebrities to get vitamin B$_{12}$ shots when they were hungover, sick, or just plain pooped; athletes sometimes use the injections to boost power. Like the other B vitamins, B$_{12}$ is often included in so-called stress-formula capsules.

Do they work?

Try not to smirk: All those pampered rock stars and athletes may have been getting needles in their bottoms for nothing. No adequate study has ever confirmed that B$_{12}$ injections fight fatigue. One small study supporting the theory that vitamin B$_{12}$ restores vitality was poorly designed and has never been replicated. Unfortunately, people plagued by chronic fatigue syndrome (CFS) aren't likely to gain much energy from vitamin B$_{12}$ supplements, either. In a 1989 study, researchers found that CFS patients who were injected with a combination of folic acid and B$_{12}$ felt no better than patients who were given a placebo preparation.

In general, there's presently little evidence that anyone who eats a balanced diet will benefit from taking high doses of vitamin B$_{12}$. However, like vitamin B$_6$ and folic acid, vitamin B$_{12}$ lowers levels of homocysteine, a substance found in the blood that's associated with an increased risk of heart disease and strokes (though folic acid may be the most effective of the three). Ongoing studies should shed light on whether reducing levels of homocysteine with vitamin therapy will prevent heart attacks and other cardiovascular problems.

What else should I know about vitamin B$_{12}$ supplements?

Vitamin B$_{12}$ is considered nontoxic, though no one should take megadoses without the supervision of a physician.

Bottom line

A balanced diet probably provides all the added B vitamins you need. If you frequently feel sluggish even though you eat right and get plenty of sleep, talk to your physician.

VITAMIN C

Also known as ascorbic acid

What is it?

Vitamin C is an antioxidant that may protect the blood and other internal fluids from damage by free radicals, which occur naturally as by-products of the way the human body uses oxygen. What's more, vitamin C is necessary for the formation of collagen, a tissue found throughout the body. It's also required for the metabolism and production of various amino acids, hormones, and other nutrients.

The recommended dietary allowance for vitamin C is 90 milligrams for adult men and 75 milligrams for women. Good sources include citrus fruits and juices, as well as peppers, berries, and broccoli. Vitamin C tablets are among the best-selling supplements in the United States. You'll often see the words *with rose hips* on bottles. Rose hips contain vitamin C and are derived from the fruit of certain species of rosebush.

Why do some people take vitamin C supplements?

Ever since Nobel laureate Linus Pauling wrote *Vitamin C and the Common Cold* in 1970, many Americans have braced themselves for winter by taking large doses of ascorbic acid. Pauling, a molecular chemist, also believed that loading up on vitamin C—up to 18 grams a day—might prevent cancer and other diseases. Some athletes take supplements containing vitamin C in the belief that it increases aerobic power and endurance.

Do they work?

Linus Pauling had his believers in the medical community, but most doctors think the brilliant scientist got a bit carried away when it came to vitamin C, particularly in regard to the common cold. A number of studies have attempted to confirm Pauling's theory during the last generation. Most determined that superdoses of vitamin C do not prevent colds. Once you catch a case of the sniffles, ascorbic acid may help limit the duration and severity of illness, but the evidence for even a mild therapeutic benefit is spotty.

The prospect of using vitamin C therapy for other conditions is being studied; here's what doctors know about a few.

Cancer

Population studies suggest that people who consume a lot of vitamin C also tend to have low rates of certain cancers, including cervical, stomach, lung, and pancreatic cancers. The stomach cancer research is particularly intriguing, since some scientists have proposed that vitamin C may prevent disease by stifling the formation of carcinogenic compounds found in some foods. But is there a cause and effect between taking high doses of vitamin C and cancer prevention? The evidence is still incomplete.

Cataracts

A study involving over fifty thousand nurses found that women who took vitamin C supplements for at least ten years were 45 percent less likely to develop this eye disease. Since eye tissue contains vitamin C, it may be that the nutrient is needed to ward off oxidative damage that leads to cataracts. But no one can say for sure whether vitamin C supplements can save vision until trials comparing them to placebos are performed.

Heart disease

Some studies have shown that people who consume large doses of vitamin C appear to reduce their risk of coronary heart disease. However, other studies suggest that simply eating the daily requirement for the nutrient may also lower your risk, while still other studies have found no connection between vitamin C levels and heart disease. More research is needed to make the argument that vitamin C is good for your heart.

Finally, there's little reason to think that vitamin C supplements will make you run any faster or longer, particularly if you eat a healthy diet. The original studies that proposed the connection were performed in Eastern European countries, where fruit and vegetables weren't always available. The athletes whose performance improved after taking vitamin C supplements may have been running on empty in the first place.

What else should I know about vitamin C supplements?

High doses may cause diarrhea and other gastrointestinal problems, as well as lead to the formation of kidney stones.

Some studies have shown that smokers have lower blood levels of vitamin C than nonsmokers, suggesting they may require greater amounts of the nutrient. If you're a dedicated five-a-day fruit and vegetable eater, you probably get plenty of vitamin C; a nonsmoking woman can get her daily dose from a single navel orange or glass of orange juice.

There's no guaranteed way to avoid catching a cold, but washing your hands with soap and water frequently to kill infectious bugs may help reduce your risk.

Bottom line

Vitamin C is an important nutrient, but its reputation as a cold-fighter is overstated. Before considering high doses of these pills, or any supplement, to prevent cancer or heart disease, examine your diet (low fat is the way to go) and talk to your physician. Proper medical screening—in the form of mammography, colonoscopy, PAP smears, and other tests—can dramatically reduce the risk of dying from cancer. And lowering cholesterol and controlling high blood pressure are essential steps to avoiding heart attacks.

VITAMIN C WITH BIOFLAVONOIDS

What is it?

You learned all about vitamin C in this book's previous entry. But if you've ever shopped for vitamin C, you may have noticed that sometimes it's sold combined with bioflavonoids. These vitamin-like substances, often identified simply as flavonoids, are found in plant foods. They aren't believed to be essential to human nutrition, but may have health benefits. Bioflavonoids come in all shapes and sizes; a few that occur in high concentrations in citrus foods (and that are often blended with vitamin C) include hesperidin, quercitrin, and rutin. Vitamin C with bioflavonoid supplements are usually sold as tablets.

Why do some people take vitamin C with bioflavonoids?

People who bruise easily sometimes use bioflavonoids to prevent and heal contusions. Special preparations containing bioflavonoids are prescribed in Europe to improve poor circulation and treat hemorrhoids, among other problems. Some sources recommend bioflavonoids for the prevention of heart disease and cancer.

> Most animals can produce their own vitamin C. Humans can't, of course, which is why we need to get it from food or supplements. We share this deficiency with other primates and, of all creatures, guinea pigs.

Does it work?

To read about vitamin C, turn to page 195. Bioflavonoids represent vast, possibly important, yet largely uncharted territory for scientists who study nutrition. Some population surveys (though not all) have found that people who eat a lot of foods rich in bioflavonoids have lower rates of heart disease, strokes, and some cancers. However, it's important to note that the findings from these studies alone don't prove much, though they suggest that eating your vegetables—as well as plenty of fruit—may turn out to be important for your health, just as your mother always told you. Furthermore, these studies looked at flavonoids in food, not isolated in supplements.

On the other hand, bioflavonoids may help specific conditions. These various plant substances are believed to strengthen capillaries, which are tiny tubes or vessels that feed blood to body tissue. Bioflavonoid products have been tested successfully for the treatment of hemorrhoids in several European studies. People plagued by this uncomfortable condition had fewer attacks when taking a special bioflavonoid preparation, which included substances found in citrus fruits. The preparation, which contained a high concentration of the bioflavonoid diosmin, appeared to make flare-ups less intense and shorter in duration, too. More research is needed, though, to understand how this product works, and whether it has broad benefits for hemorrhoid sufferers.

There has been less research on the role of bioflavonoids in improving circulation; likewise, their use to prevent or treat bruises hasn't been well studied.

What else should I know about vitamin C with bioflavonoids?

Since they occur in fruits and vegetables, it's hard to imagine that modest doses of bioflavonoids could have any harm. However, there needs to be more study of the effects of high doses of dietary supplements containing bioflavonoids. Women who take Tamoxifen, a drug used to treat and prevent breast cancer, should talk to a physician before using high doses of bioflavonoids; animal studies suggest that one in particular, known as tangeritin (a flavonoid in citrus fruit), may interfere with the drug's effectiveness. Furthermore, some bioflavonoids may act like the hormone estrogen; learn about the possible health benefits and risks of plant estrogens in the separate entry for soy, page 178.

The term *bioflavonoids* encompasses a broad spectrum of plant substances. It's often impossible to tell which ones you're buying, since labels of dietary supplements don't always specify what's inside a bottle or jar.

Bottom line

Although studies are ongoing, it's not possible at present to say which flavonoid supplements offer health benefits—or have the potential to cause harm. However, there's plenty of evidence that adding flavonoid-rich fruits and vegetables to your diet may reduce your disease risk. See the accompanying box for some ideas.

The following ten foods and beverages are flavonoid powerhouses.

Apples
Broccoli
Cabbage
Carrots
Citrus fruits
Grape juice and red wine
Onions
Peppers
Soy products (such as tofu)
Tea

VITAMIN D

Also known as known as calciferol

What is it?

Vitamin D is actually a group of related hormonelike substances, one of which is cholecalciferol, or vitamin D_3. It's often called the sunshine vitamin, since your body starts producing this important nutrient every time you take a stroll in the bright light of day. Human skin contains a vitamin precursor, known as a provitamin, which converts to vitamin D when exposed to the sun's ultraviolet rays. Vitamin D plays several roles in the body; one is to make calcium more easily absorbed into the bloodstream from the intestine.

You can also get vitamin D from your diet, although achieving the levels some experts recommend through food and drink alone isn't easy if you're trying to eat sensibly. In the United States, milk is fortified with vitamin D, as are many breakfast cereals. Fish—particularly oily ones, such as mackerel, sardines, and tuna—have modest vitamin D levels, too. But if you shun the sun, plan on eating a lot of liver, butter, and eggs to meet the minimum daily requirement. Unless, that is, you take a supplement.

Why do some people take vitamin D supplements?

To prevent osteoporosis. You probably already know that calcium is essential for strong bones. What you may not realize is that eating a calcium-rich diet and popping calcium supplements won't do you much good if your body is deficient in vitamin D.

Do they work?

Several studies have suggested that taking vitamin D supplements may reduce bone loss and the risk of broken bones in the elderly. Vitamin D deficiency is surprisingly common in the United States, particularly in the northern states during the winter—even among apparently healthy people. Boston University researchers studied blood samples from nearly three hundred patients hospitalized for various reasons and found that almost 60 percent of them had insufficient levels of vitamin D. Even people who took multivitamins were included among those lacking in this critical nutrient.

Another study, also conducted in the Boston area—where venturing outdoors during the chilly winters can lose its appeal—found that elderly women who fracture their hips also tend to have low levels of vitamin D. Given the mounting evidence, the Institute of Medicine has determined that an adequate intake for people fifty-one to seventy years old is 400 IU of vitamin D per day. (This amount is sometimes noted as 10 μg.) After age seventy, the recommended adequate intake is 600 IU (or 15 μg), although during the cold months 800 IU might be necessary. The best advice is to consult your physician, since people who spend a lot of time in the sun may make adequate vitamin D on their own.

The liver and kidneys convert vitamin D_3 to a more active substance called calcitrol. Some laboratory studies suggest that calcitrol may inhibit the growth of tumors; clinical studies are under way to determine if it's beneficial in fighting cancer.

What else should I know about vitamin D supplements?

Very high doses of vitamin D—in the range of 50,000 IU daily—can be toxic. The body absorbs too much calcium and phosphorus, causing excessive thirst, stomach upset, and depression. Over time, getting too much vitamin D could cause kidney stones.

A typical multivitamin provides 400 IU of vitamin D. If you're under fifty and get outside every day for at least fifteen minutes (without sunscreen, which blocks UV rays), you may not need vitamin D supplements. A complete bone-health regimen should include adequate calcium; unless you consume a lot of dairy products, you should consider adding a calcium supplement.

Bottom line

Vitamin D may have an important role in preventing osteoporosis. Talk to your physician about how, and if, these supplements should be included in a regimen to promote bone health. While you're at it, be sure to discuss other important interventions that may prevent osteoporosis, including calcium and—for women who have reached menopause—estrogen replacement therapy.

VITAMIN E

Sometimes labeled as alpha-tocopherol

What is it?

Vitamin E is a family of related substances, but the name usually refers to the one that's most important to humans, known as alpha-tocopherol.

Vitamin E is an antioxidant that protects the membranes of cells from damage by free radicals that may lead to heart disease and certain cancers.

Vitamin E deficiency is rare and most Americans easily meet the recommended daily requirement for vitamin E. Some rich sources include vegetable oils, whole grains, nuts, and leafy green vegetables. Supplements are usually sold in the form of gelatin capsules.

Why do some people use vitamin E supplements?

Many Americans take the vitamin on doctor's orders, since it has gained a reputation for reducing the risk of cardiovascular disease. But vitamin E has been studied for the prevention and treatment of several conditions including Alzheimer's disease, some cancers, diabetes, cataracts, and AIDS. What's more, so-called all-natural Viagra alternatives that promise to boost a man's sexual potency often contain vitamin E.

Do they work?

In theory, yes. In the real world—well, that's not so clear. Vitamin E shines in the lab, where test-tube studies have shown that it prevents LDL cholesterol from being oxidized (which makes it "bad," and capable of clogging arteries). Scientists have also shown that vitamin E prevents disclike substances in the blood called platelets from clumping together to form clots that lead to heart attacks. Furthermore, vitamin E dilates blood vessels, allowing for freer flow of blood.

Interest in vitamin E's promise for preventing heart attacks began when a few observational studies turned up evidence that people who use the supplements tend to have low rates of cardiovascular disease. Americans have responded by making it one of the most popular single vitamins sold in this country. However, it's possible that people who use vitamin E may also have other healthy habits that reduce their risk of heart disease—they may exercise a lot, for instance, or eat healthier foods. To find out whether vitamin E safeguards the heart, scientists have compared groups of subjects given the supplement with similar groups of people who were given inactive placebo pills. Unfortunately, no clear answer has emerged from these studies.

For example, Canadian researchers followed a group of over ninety-five hundred people who were at high risk for heart disease for more than four years. They gave half the group 400 IU of vitamin E every day; the other half received sugar pills. At the study's conclusion, the people taking high doses of vitamin E were just as likely to have suffered a heart attack or stroke as those taking placebos. Yet, earlier research suggested that a daily dose of 400 or 800 IU of vitamin E decreased the risk of both fatal and nonfatal heart attacks in men with coronary artery disease. These conflicting results have yielded more questions than answers for scientists.

Vitamin E may one day prove to be an effective means of preventing prostate cancer, the most common form of the disease found in American men besides skin cancer. Although improved screening methods have increased the ability to detect this cancer early, when it responds better to treatment, finding a way to prevent the disease from developing in the first place would save countless lives. A Finnish study found that the risk of prostate cancer among male tobacco smokers who were given 50 IU of vitamin E a day for six years dropped by 32 percent. Encouraged by this data, scientists in the United States have launched another large study (called the SELECT trial) comparing vitamin E and another suspected prostate cancer fighter, selenium, with a placebo. (Read about selenium on page 173).

To date, there's not enough evidence to recommend the use of vitamin E to prevent or treat other conditions.

What else should I know about vitamin E supplements?

Vitamin E is generally considered safe, with a caveat or two. One large study found that taking supplemental vitamin E may increase the risk of death from strokes caused by bleeding in the brain among people who have high blood pressure. The increased risk was small, but if you're considering taking vitamin E, consult your physician first, especially if you have hypertension or if you take any type of blood-thinning medication or drug intended to suppress the immune system.

Many vitamin E supplements contain a synthetic form of the vitamin that's made from petrochemicals—even though the labels may say "natural." Truly natural vitamin E, made from vegetable oil, is about 50 percent more potent than the synthetic version. To buy all-natural vitamin

E, read the ingredient list and look for d-alpha-tocopherol. (Synthetic vitamin E may be identified as dl-alpha-tocopherol.) However, it's worth noting that the synthetic form of vitamin E was used in the study mentioned earlier that found a decreased risk of prostate cancer.

Bottom line

Vitamin E may play a role in preventing cardiovascular disease and prostate cancer, but the scientific evidence remains inconclusive. Talk to a physician before taking vitamin E, since it has a small risk of complications and may interact with some medications.

VITAMIN K

What is it?

A Danish scientist discovered that when chickens had too little of this substance, they bled excessively. That's why he called it the koagulations vitamin, since it causes blood to clot, or coagulate—which is exactly what you want to happen when you cut your finger or have a nose bleed. Now known simply as vitamin K, this nutrient may also be critical for healthy bones, especially in developing fetuses.

Vitamin K is found in many foods, especially leafy green vegetables. Intestinal bacteria manufacture the vitamin, too. Some—though not all—multivitamins contain a dose of vitamin K.

Why do some people take vitamin K supplements?

Vitamin K is often included in so-called bone formula pills and preparations used by consumers concerned about osteoporosis.

Do they work?

Vitamin K has several well-established medical uses. It's sometimes administered to newborn infants to improve their blood's clotting ability, since they have low levels of vitamin K for a few days after birth. Physicians also use vitamin K to counteract the blood-thinning effects of medications such as warfarin.

On the other hand, researchers are still trying to understand whether vitamin K has a role in treating other medical conditions, particularly osteoporosis. Two large studies published in the *American Journal of Clinical Nutrition* have shown that elderly men and women whose diets contain very little of this nutrient were more likely to fracture bones than people who eat lots of foods rich in vitamin K. The key word here is *eat*. These studies didn't take into consideration the use of supplements, but focused on how much vitamin K people got from food sources. Furthermore, this research doesn't prove conclusively that high vitamin K intake prevented broken bones; people who consume large amounts of this vitamin may have other healthy habits that safeguard them from osteoporosis. In short, much more research is needed to show that high doses of vitamin K benefit bones.

What else should I know about vitamin K supplements?

People who take anticoagulant drugs, such as warfarin, may need them to prevent potential blood clots in the lungs, heart, and other organs. High levels of vitamin K could interfere with the action of these drugs.

Bottom line

Adequate studies demonstrating the safety and therapeutic value of vitamin K supplements have yet to be performed. It's easy to get sufficient amounts of this nutrient from a balanced diet. Vitamin K should not be used without a physician's guidance.

YOHIMBE

Scientific name: *Pausinystalia yohimbe*

What is it?

The yohimbe tree grows in West Africa. Its bark contains a compound called yohimbine. A drug containing yohimbine, sold under several brand names, is available by prescription in the United States. However, dried yohimbe bark is also available as a dietary supplement, in capsule, tablet, powder, or liquid form.

Why do some people take yohimbe supplements?

Yohimbe has long been considered an aphrodisiac in Africa. In this country, it's sold in health food stores and on the Internet, and marketed to men with erectile dysfunction (ED) as a "natural" alternative to Viagra (often using sly, suggestive language). Some athletes use yohimbe as a performance-enhancing supplement, too.

Do they work?

Yohimbe bark hasn't been well studied for the treatment of erectile dysfunction. However, research has been conducted on the prescription drug yohimbine for that purpose. In theory, yohimbine may help a man achieve and sustain an erection through several mechanisms, particularly by increasing blood flow to the penis. In the real world, though, yohimbine's effectiveness is a matter of debate. Some studies have shown it to have modest benefits, while others have found yohimbine to be no better than a sugar pill.

But even if you take the optimistic view that the drug yohimbine works for some men with erectile dysfunction, that doesn't necessarily mean that commercially available yohimbe bark will, too. The amount of active ingredient in herbal preparations isn't regulated in this country, and some products may not contain enough yohimbine to exert a drug-like effect. In fact, a 1995 analysis of twenty-six commercial yohimbe products found that nine contained no yohimbine, while eight had only trace amounts.

Despite claims made by sellers of sports supplements, there's no definitive evidence that yohimbe makes athletes faster or stronger. And reports that the herb will make your body "burn fat" are based on flimsy evidence.

What else should I know about yohimbe supplements?

A number of potential side effects have been linked to the drug yohimbine, including dizziness, headaches, anxiety, elevated blood pressure, tremors, nausea, and vomiting. There have also been reports of users who developed eczema and whose kidneys failed. Anyone with hypertension, diabetes, and heart or liver disease should avoid both the drug and the herb. Men given prescriptions for yohimbine are ordered not to consume the following foods and beverages: cheese, chocolate, aged meats, beer, and red wine. Finally, yohimbine may interact with a long list of medications.

Bottom line

Because yohimbe supplements may contain the active drug yohimbine—in unpredictable doses—it should be considered particularly dangerous. Erectile dysfunction can be a symptom of many serious conditions, which is why it should be evaluated by a physician, who can discuss the use of Viagra and other treatment options.

ZINC

What is it?

Zinc is a trace mineral, which is an inorganic chemical your body needs, but only in tiny amounts. However, even though you carry just a few grams of zinc, it's vital for the formation of dozens of enzymes that govern a long list of bodily functions. Zinc is necessary for the growth and development of bones and reproductive organs. It's involved in the breakdown of carbohydrates and production of proteins. Proper levels of zinc are needed for wound healing, eye pigment, sperm production, and a healthy immune system. Even your taste buds depend on zinc.

Heavy drinking can cause zinc deficiency, as can an inherited disorder called acrodermatitis enteropathica. In rare cases, vegetarians don't get enough of the mineral since the best sources include meat, eggs, and seafood. Zinc is sold in lozenge and pill form, and you'll almost always find the mineral in multivitamins.

Why do some people use zinc supplements?

Zinc lozenges have become hugely popular with cold sufferers in recent years. Zinc supplements have also been used to treat a number of other conditions, including acne, enlarged prostate, night blindness, and male infertility.

Do they work?

Although some scientists believe that zinc can banish a case of the sniffles, the evidence remains shaky. A much-publicized study at the Cleveland Clinic in 1996 compared zinc lozenges with placebo pills. People who began taking zinc at the onset of cold symptoms quit coughing sooner and their nasal congestion cleared up faster than in people who were given placebos. A few other small studies of zinc users have come up with similar results.

But for every glowing scientific report suggesting that zinc lozenges are the natural cure for the common cold, there seems to be another calling them worthless. A review of the existing research in the *Journal of Nutrition* in 2000 determined that there is still no clear proof that zinc is worth your money when you're battling a scratchy throat and runny nose.

There's little evidence that zinc supplements are a good choice for treating any of the other conditions mentioned, unless they're caused by zinc deficiency, which must be diagnosed—and treated—by a physician.

What else should I know about zinc supplements?

Few people become addicted to the taste of zinc lozenges. (In fact, subjects have been known to drop out of zinc studies with, pardon the pun, a bad taste in their mouths.) Zinc can also cause nausea and vomiting. There are reports that excess zinc intake may cause blood levels of both the mineral copper and HDL ("good") cholesterol to drop. High levels of the mineral could also interfere with drugs intended to suppress the immune system, including cyclosporine and the corticosteroids. By the way, the accuracy of so-called hair analysis tests, which purportedly measure levels of zinc and other minerals in the body, is questionable.

Avoiding exposure to the rhinovirus germs that cause most colds is difficult, but frequent hand washing can't hurt.

Bottom line

Zinc is an important mineral, but supplements should only be used under the supervision of a physician.

NOTES

Journal citations follow this format:
Name of Journal
Year of Publication
Volume Number
Pages

INTRODUCTION

1. *Archives of Family Medicine*, 1998; 7:523–36.
2. *Archives of Internal Medicine*, 1998; 158:2192–99.
3. *Archives of Internal Medicine*, 1998; 158:2200–11.
4. *Critical Reviews in Food Sciences and Nutrition*, 1999; 39:317–28.
5. *Journal of the American Pharmaceutical Association*, 2000; 40:234–42.
6. *Psychosomatic Medicine*, 1999; 61:712–28.
7. *Sports Medicine*, 1999; 27:97–110.

ACIDOPHILUS

1. *Journal of the American Medical Association*, 1996; 275:870–86.
2. *American Journal of Clinical Nutrition*, 2000; 71:405–11.
3. *Journal of Nutrition*, 2000; 130:396S–402S.
4. *Journal of the American College of Nutrition*, 1999; 18:43–50.

ALFALFA

1. *British Journal of Medicine*, 1997; 78:325–34.
2. *Atherosclerosis*, 1987; 65:173–79.
3. *Lancet*, 1981; 1:615.

ALOE VERA

1. *Gut*, 1993; 34:1099–101.

ALPHA-LIPOIC ACID

1. *Diabetes*, 1997; 46:62S–66S.
2. *Diabetic Medicine*, 1999; 16:1040–43.
3. *Free Radical Biology & Medicine*, 1999; 27:309–14.
4. *Free Radical Biology & Medicine*, 1995; 19:227–50.
5. *Free Radical Biology & Medicine*, 1999; 27:1114–21.

AMINO ACID AND PROTEIN SUPPLEMENTS

1. *Critical Reviews in Food Science and Nutrition*, 1999; 39:317–28.
2. *Sports Medicine*, 1999; 27:97–110.

ANTIOXIDANT FORMULAS

1. *New England Journal of Medicine*, 1994; 330:1080–81.
2. *American Journal of Clinical Nutrition*, 2000; 72:637S–46S.

ARGININE

1. *Circulation*, 1996; 93:2135–41.
2. *Journal of the American College of Cardiology*, 2000; 35:706–13.
3. *Circulation*, 1998; 97:2123–28.
4. *Heart*, 1999; 81:512–27.
5. *Circulation*, 2000; 101:2160–64.
6. *Journal of the American College of Cardiology*, 1998; 32:1336–44.
7. *Vascular Medicine*, 2000; 5:11–19.
8. *BJU International*, 1999; 83:269–73.
9. *Urologia Internationalis*, 1999; 63:220–23.

BARLEY GRASS

1. *Journal of the American Dietetic Association*, 1994; 94:65–70.
2. *Journal of the American Dietetic Association*, 1993; 93:881–85.

BEE POLLEN

1. *Journal of Sport Medicine and Physical Fitness*, 1978; 18:221–26.
2. *British Journal of Sports Medicine*, 1982; 16:142–45.
3. *British Journal of Urology*, 1989; 64:496–99.
4. *Prostate*, 1998; 37:187–93.

BETA CAROTENE

1. *New England Journal of Medicine*, 1994; 330:1029–35.
2. *New England Journal of Medicine*, 1996; 334:1145–49.
3. *New England Journal of Medicine*, 1996; 334:1150–55.
4. *New England Journal of Medicine*, 1994; 331:141–47.
5. *New England Journal of Medicine*, 1990; 323:789–95.
6. *Journal of the American Medical Association*, 1996; 275:699–703.
7. *Journal of the American Medical Association*, 1996; 275:693–98.

BILBERRY

1. *Eye*, 1998; 12:967–69.
2. *Eye*, 1999; 13:734–36.

BIOTIN

1. *Cutis*, 1993; 51:303–05.
2. *Journal of the American Academy of Dermatology*, 1990; 23:1127–32.

BLACK COHOSH

1. *Journal of the American Pharmaceutical Association*, 2000; 40:234–42.
2. *Menopause*, 1998; 5:250.
3. *Journal of Clinical Oncology*, 2000; 19:2739–45.

CALCIUM

1. *New England Journal of Medicine*, 1993; 328:460–64.
2. *New England Journal of Medicine*, 1999; 340;101–07.
3. *New England Journal of Medicine*, 1992; 327:1637–42.

CARNITINE

1. *Sports Medicine*, 1996; 2:109–32.
2. *International Journal of Sport Nutrition and Exercise Metabolism*, 2000; 10:199–207.
3. *Clinical Pharmacology, Therapy, and Toxicology*, 1985; 23:569–72.
4. *Drugs in Experimental Clinical Research*, 1991; 7:225–35.
5. *American Heart Journal*, 2000; 139:120S–23S.

CAT'S CLAW

1. *Journal of Ethnopharmacology*, 1999; 64:109–15.

CAYENNE

1. *Digestive Diseases and Sciences*, 1995; 40:580.

CHAMOMILE

1. *Archives of General Psychiatry*, 1998; 55:1033–44.

CHILDREN'S VITAMINS

1. *Pediatrics*, 1997; 100:E4. Online. Internet. 18 Feb. 2001. (www. pediatrics.org)

CHITOSAN

1. *European Journal of Clinical Nutrition*, 1999; 53:379–81.

CHOLINE

1. *Clinical Neuropharmacology*, 1993;16: 540–49.
2. *Nutrition Reviews*, 1994; 52:327–39.
3. *Medicine and Science in Sports and Exercise*, 1995; 27:668–73.
4. *International Journal of Sports Nutrition, Exercise, and Metabolism*, 2000; 10:170–81.

CHONDROITIN

1. *Journal of the American Medical Association*, 2000; 283:1469–75.
2. *Journal of Rheumatology*, 2000; 27:205–11.

CHROMIUM

1. *Physician and Sportsmedicine*, 1997; 25. Online. Internet. 15 Feb. 2001. (www.physsportsmed.com/issues/1997/06jun/armsey.htm)
2. *Sports Medicine*, 1999; 27:97–110.
3. *Clinical Diabetes*, 1997; 15. Online. Internet. 18 Feb. 2001. (www.diabetes.org/clinicaldiabetes/v15m1j-f97/pg6.htm)
4. American Diabetes Association, Position Statement, Nutrition Recommendations and Principles for People with Diabetes Mellitus. Online. Internet. 18 Feb. 2001. (www.diabetes.org/diabetescare/supplement/s16.htm)

COENZYME Q$_{10}$

1. *Clinical Investigations*, 1993; 71:134S–6S.
2. *Annals of Internal Medicine*, 2000; 132:636–40.
3. *American Journal of Clinical Nutrition*, 1997; 65:503–07.

CRANBERRY EXTRACT

1. *Journal of the American Medical Association*, 1994; 271:751–54.
2. *Journal of Family Practice*, 197; 45:167–68.
3. *Western Journal of Medicine*, 1999; 171:195–98.

CREATINE

1. *Journal of the American Dietetic Association*, 1997; 97:765–70.
2. *Nutrition Reviews*, 1999; 57:45–50.
3. *British Journal of Sports Medicine*, 1996; 30:276–81.

DHEA

1. *Critical Reviews in Food Science and Nutrtion*, 1999; 39:317–28.
2. *Medicine & Science in Sports & Exercise*, 1999; 31:1788–92.
3. *Journal of Clinical Pharmacology*, 1999; 39:327–48.
4. *Urology*, 1999; 53:590–95.
5. *Archives of Internal Medicine*, 2000; 160:2193–98.
6. *Rheumatic Disease Clinics of North America*, 2000; 26:349–62.
7. *New England Journal of Medicine*, 1999; 341:1013–20.

DONG QUAI

1. *Fertility and Sterility*, 1997; 68:981–86.
2. *Pharmacotherapy*, 1999; 19:870–76.

ECHINACEA

1. *Archives of Family Medicine*, 1998; 7:527–28.
2. *Archives of Family Medicine*, 1998; 7:541–45.
3. *American Journal of Medicine*, 1999; 106:138–43.

ENZYME FORMULAS

1. *Scandanavian Journal of Gastroenterology*, 1990; 25:298–301.
2. *Annals of Internal Medicine*, 2000; 132:680

EPHEDRA

1. *International Journal of Obesity*, 1987; 11:163–68.
2. *International Journal of Obesity*, 1992; 16:269–77.
3. *Drugs*, 1999; 57:883–904.
4. *New England Journal of Medicine*, 2000; 343:1833–88.
5. *American Journal of Health-system Pharmacy*, 2000; 57:963–69.

6. *International Journal of Obesity and Related Metabolic Disorders,* 2001; 25:316–24.

ESSENTIAL FATTY ACIDS
No studies cited.

EVENING PRIMROSE OIL
1. *British Journal of Rheumatology,* 1991; 30:370–72.
2. *Annals of Internal Medicine,* 1993; 119:867-73.
3. *American Journal of Clinical Nutrition,* 2000; 71:352S–56S.
4. *Journal of the American College of Nutrition,* 2000; 19:3–12.
5. *Journal of the American Pharmaceutical Association,* 2000; 40:234–42.

EYEBRIGHT
No studies cited.

FEVERFEW
1. *Journal of the American Medical Association,* 1992; 267:64–69.
2. *Lancet,* 1988; 2:189–92.
3. *Annals of Rheumatic Diseases,* 1989; 48:547–49.

FIBER SUPPLEMENTS
1. *New England Journal of Medicine,* 1999; 340:169–76.
2. *New England Journal of Medicine,* 2000; 342:1149–55.
3. *New England Journal of Medicine,* 2000; 342:1156–62.
4. *Journal of the American Medical Association,* 1999; 282:1539–46.

FISH OIL
1. *American Journal of Clinical Nutrition,* 1980; 33:2657–61.
2. *New England Journal of Medicine,* 1995; 332:977–82.
3. *European Journal of Clinical Nutrition,* 1999; 53:585–90.

4. *American Journal of Epidemiololgy,* 2000; 151:999–1006.
5. *Annals of Internal Medicine,* 1999; 130:554–62.
6. *Circulation,* 1992; 85:950–56.
7. *Journal of American College of Cardiology,* 1999; 33:1619–26.
8. *Journal of American College of Cardiology,* 1995; 25:1492–98.
9. *Arthritis and Rheumatism,* 1990; 33:810–20.
10. *British Journal of Rheumatology,* 1993; 32:982–89.
11. *Arthritis and Rheumatism,* 1995; 38:1107–14.
12. *Journal of the American Medical Association,* 1998; 279:23–28.

FLAXSEED

1. *American Journal of Clinical Nutrition,* 1999; 69:395–402.
2. *Rheumatology International,* 1995; 14:231–34.

FOLIC ACID

1. *Lancet,* 1991; 338:131–37.
2. *New England Journal of Medicine,* 1992; 327:1832–35.
3. *Journal of the American Medical Association,* 1992; 268:877–81.
4. *Journal of the American Medical Association,* 1995; 274:1049–57.

GARLIC

1. *Journal of Hypertension,* 1994; 12:463–68.
2. *American Journal of Clinical Nutrition,* 1996; 64:866–70S.
3. *Journal of the Royal College of Physicians of London,* 1996; 30:329–34.
4. *Archives of Internal Medicine,* 1998; 158:1189–94.
5. *Journal of the American Medical Association,* 1998; 279:1900–02.
6. *Journal of the American College of Cardiology,* 2000; 35:321–26.
7. *Annals of Internal Medicine,* 2000; 133:420–29.
8. *Atherosclerosis,* 2001; 154:213–20.

GINGER

1. *Acta Oto-laryngolica,* 1988; 105:45–49.
2. *Lancet,* 1982; 1:655–57.

3. *Pharmacology,* 1991; 42:111–20.
4. *Anaesthesia,* 1993; 48:715–17.
5. *Anaesthesia and Intensive Care,* 1995; 23:449–52.
6. *Anaesthesia,* 1998; 53:506–10.

GINKGO

1. *Journal of the American Medical Association,* 1997; 278:1327–32.
2. *Current Medical Research and Opinion,* 1991; 12:350–55.
3. *Drugs,* 2000; 59:1057–70.
4. *Journal of Sex and Marital Therapy,* 1998; 24:139–43.
5. *American Journal of Psychiatry,* 2000; 157:836–37.

GINSENG

1. *Sports Medicine,* 2000; 29:113–33.
2. *Archives of Internal Medicine,* 2000; 160:1009–13.
3. *Journal of the American Dietetic Association,* 1997; 97:1110–15.
4. *Journal of the American College of Nutrition,* 1998; 17:462–66.
5. *Drugs and Experimental Clinical Research,* 1996; 22:65–72.
6. *Cancer Causes and Control,* 2000; 11:565–76.
7. *International Journal of Impotence Research,* 1995; 7:181–86.

GLUCOSAMINE

Journal of the American Medical Association, 2000; 283:1469–75.

GOLDENSEAL

1. *Immunology Letters,* 1999; 68:391–95.
2. *British Medical Journal (Clinical Resident Education),* 1985;
   291:1601–05.
3. *Journal of Infectious Diseases,* 1987; 155:979–84.

GRAPE SEED EXTRACT

1. *Atherosclerosis,* 1999; 142:139–49.
2. *Journal of Clinical Pharmacy and Therapeutics,* 1998; 23:385–89.

3. *Carcinogenesis*, 1999; 20:1737–45.
4. *Molecular Cell Biochemistry*, 1999; 196:99–108.

GREEN TEA EXTRACT

1. *American Journal of Clinical Nutrition*, 2000; 7:1698S–1702S.
2. *Critical Reviews in Food Science and Nutrition*, 1997; 37:771–85.
3. *American Journal of Clinical Nutrition*, 1999; 70:1040–45.
4. *New England Journal of Medicine*, 2001; 344:632–36.

GUARANA

1. *Alternative Medicine Alert*, 1999; 2:67–70.
2. *Journal of Pharmacy and Pharmacology*, 1992; 44:769–71.

HAWTHORN

1. *Western Journal of Medicine*, 1999; 171:191–94.
2. *American Family Physician*, 2000; 62:1325–30.

HORSE CHESTNUT EXTRACT

1. *Archives of Dermatology*, 1998; 134:1356–60.
2. *Lancet*, 1996; 347:292–94.

INOSITOL

1. *New England Journal of Medicine*, 1992; 326:1233–39.
2. *American Journal of Psychiatry*, 1995; 152:792–94.
3. *Biological Psychiatry*, 1999; 45:270–73.
4. *American Journal of Psychiatry*, 1995; 152:1084–86.
5. *American Journal of Psychiatry*, 1996; 153:1219–21.
6. *Journal of Psychiatric Research*, 1997; 31:489–95.

IRON

1. *Journal of Applied Physiology*, 2000; 88:1103–11.

KAVA

1. *Journal of Clinical Psychopharmacology*, 2000; 20:84–89.
2. *Western Journal of Medicine*, 1999; 171:195–98.

KELP

1. *Journal of Allergy Clinical Immunology*, 1995; 75:138.

LECITHIN

1. *American Journal of Clinical Nutrition*, 1989; 49:266–68.
2. *European Journal of Clinical Nutrition*, 1998; 52:419–24.
3. *Neurology*, 1981; 31:1552–54.
4. *Archives of Neurology*, 1983; 40:527–28.
5. *Journal of Neural Transmission*, 1987; 24:279S–86S.

LICORICE

1. *Gut*, 1971; 12:449–51.
2. *British Medical Journal*, 1977; 2:1123.
3. *Gut*, 1978; 19:779–82.
4. *New England Journal of Medicine*, 1999; 341:1158.
5. *Anticancer Research*, 2000; 20:2653–58.

LUTEIN

1. *Journal of the American Medical Association*, 1994; 272:1413–20.
2. *American Journal of Clinical Nutrition*, 1999; 70:517–24.
3. *American Journal of Clinical Nutrition*, 2000; 71:575–82.

LYSINE

1. *Journal of the American College of Nutrition*, 1997; 16:7–21.
2. *Lancet*, 1978; 2:942.
3. *Dermatologica*, 1987; 175:183–90.
4. *Archives of Dermatology*, 1985; 121:167–68.
5. *Cutis*, 1984; 34:366–73.
6. *Acta Dermato-venereologica*, 1980; 60:85–87.

MAGNESIUM

1. *Headache*, 1996; 36:154–60.
2. *Cephalalgia*, 1996; 16:257–63.
3. *Cephalalgia*, 1996; 16:436–40.
4. *Lancet*, 1991; 337:757–60.
5. *Journal of the American College of Nutrition*, 2000; 19:374–82.
6. *Magnesium Research*, 1997; 10:149–56.

MELATONIN

1. *British Medical Journal*, 1989; 298:705–07.
2. *Biological Psychiatry*, 1992; 32:705–11.
3. *American Journal of Psychiatry*, 1999; 156:1392–96.
4. *Biological Psychiatry*, 1993; 33:526–30.
5. *Clinical Pharmacology and Therapeutics*, 1995; 57:552–58.
6. *American Journal of Medicine*, 1999; 107:432–36.
7. *Lancet*, 1995; 346:541–44.
8. *Journal of Sleep Research*, 1996; 5:61–65.
9. *Sleep*, 2000; 23: 663–69.

MILK THISTLE

1. *Scandinavian Journal of Gastroenterology*, 1982; 17:517–21.
2. *Journal of Hepatology*, 1989; 9:105–13.
3. *Revista Medica Chile*, 1992; 120:1370–75.
4. *Journal of Hepatology*, 1998; 28:615–21.
5. *Archives of Family Medicine*, 1998; 7:523–36.

MSM

1. *Cryobiology*, 23:14–27.

MULTIMINERALS/TRACE MINERALS

No studies cited.

MULTIVITAMINS

1. *Journal of the American Geriatric Society*, 1987; 35:302–36.
2. *Journal of the American College of Nutrition*, 2000; 19:613–21.
3. *Annals of Internal Medicine*, 1998; 129:517–24.
4. *American Journal of Epidemiology*, 2000; 152:149–62.
5. *Annals of Epidemiology*, 2000; 10:125–34.

N-ACETYL CYSTEINE

1. *European Journal of Respiratory Diseases*, 1983; 64:405–15.
2. *British Journal of Diseases of the Chest*, 1987; 81:341–48.
3. *Circulation*, 1992; 85:143–49.
4. *Journal of Clinical Investigation*, 1994; 94:2468–74.
5. *Journal of Pediatrics*, 1994; 124:229–33.
6. *Respiratory Medicine*, 1994; 88:531–35.
7. *Journal of the American College of Cardiology*, 1997; 29:941–47.

NIACIN

1. *Archives of Internal Medicine*, 1994; 154:1586–95.
2. *American Journal of Cardiology*, 2000; 85:1100–05.
3. *American Heart Journal*, 1999; 138:1082–87.
4. *Journal of the American Medical Association*, 1994; 271:672–77.

PANTETHINE AND PANTOTHENIC ACID

1. *Current Therapeutic Research*, 1983; 34:383–90.
2. *International Journal of Clinical Pharmacology, Therapy, and Toxicology*, 1986; 24:630–37.
3. *Minerva Medica*, 1990; 81:475–79.
4. *Practitioner*, 1980; 224:208–11.

PAPAYA AND PAPAIN

1. *Dermatology*, 1997; 194:364–66.

PC-SPES

1. *New England Journal of Medicine*, 1998; 339:785–91.
2. *Journal of Clinical Oncology*, 2000; 18:3595–603.

PHOSPHORUS

1. *Medicine and Science in Sports and Exercise*, 1990; 22:250–56.
2. *International Journal of Sports Nutrition*, 1992; 2:20–47.

POTASSIUM

1. *Journal of the American Medical Association*, 1997; 277:1624–32.
2. *New England Journal of Medicine*,1997; 336:1117–24.
3. *Hypertension*, 1998; 31:131–38.

PRENATAL VITAMINS

1. *American Journal of Epidemiology*, 1997; 146:134–41.
2. *International Journal of Cancer Supplement*, 1998; 11:17–22.

PYCNOGENOL

1. *Free Radical Biological Medicine*, 1999; 27: 704–24.
2. *Thrombosis Research*, 1999; 95:155–61.

PYGEUM

1. *Current Medical Research and Opinion*, 1998; 14:127–39.
2. *Wiener Klinische Wochenschrift*, 1990; 102:667–73.
3. *Urology*, 1999; 54:473–78.

PYRUVATE

1. *American Journal of Clinical Nutrition*, 1992; 55:771–76.
2. *Nutrition*, 1999; 15:337–40.
3. *International Journal of Sports Nutrition*, 1999; 9:146–65.
4. *American Journal of Clinical Nutrition*, 1994; 59:423–27.

RED YEAST RICE

1. *American Journal of Clinical Nutrition*, 1999; 69:231–36.
2. *Allergy*, 1999; 54:1330–31.

RIBOFLAVIN

1. *Neurology*, 1998; 50:466–70.
2. *Ophthalmology*, 2000; 107:450–56.

ROYAL JELLY

1. *Experientia*, 1995; 51:927–35.

SAINT-JOHN'S-WORT

1. *British Medical Journal*, 1996; 313:253–58.
2. *Archives of Internal Medicine*, 2000; 160:152–56.
3. *Clinical Therapeutics*, 2000; 22:411–19.
4. *Journal of the American Medical Association*, 2001; 285:1978–86.

SAMe

1. *Acta Neurologica Scandinavica*, 1994; 154:7S–14S.
2. *Acta Psychiatrica Scandinavica*, 1990; 81:432–36.
3. *American Journal of Psychiatry*, 1990; 147:591–95.
4. *Acta Neurologica Scandinavica*, 1994; 154:19S–26S.
5. *Journal of Pharmacology and Experimental Therapeutics*, 1979; 209:323–26.
6. *Scandinavian Journal of Rheumatology*, 1997; 26:206–11.
7. *American Journal of Medicine*, 1987; 83:81–83.
8. *Journal of Hepatology*, 2000; 32:113S–28S.

SAW PALMETTO

1. *Journal of the American Medical Association*, 1998; 280:1604–09.
2. *Journal of Urology*, 2000; 163:1408–12.
3. *Journal of Urology*, 2000; 163:1451–56.

SELENIUM

1. *Journal of the American Medical Association*, 1996; 276:1957–63 (published erratum in *Journal of the American Medical Association*, 1997; 277:1520).
2. *Journal of the National Cancer Institute*, 1993; 85:1483–92.

SHARK CARTILAGE

1. *Science*, 1983; 221:1185–87.
2. *Acta Oncologica*, 1998; 37:441–45.
3. *Journal of Clinical Oncology*, 1998; 16:3649–55.

SIBERIAN GINSENG

1. *Medicine and Science in Sports and Exercise*, 1996; 28:482–89.
2. *Arzneimittelforschung*, 1987; 37:1193–96.
3. *Lancet*, 2000; 355:134–38.

SOY AND SOY ISOFLAVONES

1. *New England Journal of Medicine*, 1995; 333:276–82.
2. *American Journal of Clinical Nutrition*, 2000; 71:1077–84.
3. *Journal of Clinical Endocrinology and Metabolism*, 1999; 84:4017–24.
4. *American Journal of Clinical Nutrition*, 1998; 68:1375S–79S.
6. *Menopause*, 2000; 7:215–29.
7. *Journal of the American Medical Association*, 2001; 285:1482–88.

SPIRULINA

1. *Journal of the American Medical Association*, 1982; 248:3096–97.
2. *American Journal of Clinical Nutrition*, 1991; 53:695–97.

THIAMIN

1. *Journal of Geriatric Psychiatry and Neurology*, 1993; 6:222–29.
2. *Metabolic Brain Disease*, 1996; 11:89–94.
3. *Psychopharmacology*, 1997; 129:66–71.

VALERIAN

1. *Pharmacology Biochemistry and Behavior,* 1982; 17:65–71.
2. *Pharmacology Biochemistry and Behavior,* 1989; 32:1065–66.
3. *Planta Medica,* 1985; 144–48.

VANADYL SULFATE

1. *Critical Reviews in Food Science and Nutrition,* 1999; 39:317–28.
2. *Sports Medicine,* 1999; 27:97–110.
3. *Metabolism,* 1996; 45:1130–35.
4. *Journal of Clinical Investigation,* 1995; 95:2501–09.
5. *Diabetes,* 1996; 45:659–66.
6. *Metabolism,* 2000; 49:1130–35.

VITAMIN A

1. *Journal of Clinical Oncology,* 1994; 12:2060–65.
2. *Journal of the National Cancer Institute,* 2000; 92:977–86.

VITAMIN B COMPLEX

1. *Journal of the Royal Society of Medicine,* 1999; 92:183–85.

VITAMIN B_6

1. *Journal of the American Medical Association,* 1998; 279:359–64.
2. *New England Journal of Medicine,* 1983; 309:445–48.

VITAMIN B_{12}

1. *New England Journal of Medicine,* 2000; 342:981.
2. *Journal of the American Medical Association,* 1989; 261:1920–23.
3. *British Journal of Nutrition,* 1973; 30:277–83.
4. *Family Medicine,* 1991; 23:506–59.
5. *Medical Hypotheses,* 1991; 34:131–40.
6. *International Journal of Geriatric Psychiatry,* 1998; 13:611–16.

VITAMIN C

1. *Journal of the American Medical Association*, 1975; 231:1038–42.
2. *Journal of the American Medical Association*, 1975; 231:1073–79.
3. *Journal of the American Medical Association*, 1975; 234:149.
4. *Journal of the American Medical Association*, 1977; 237:248–51.
5. *British Medical Journal*, 1992; 305:335–39.
6. *Lancet*, 1999; 354:2048.

VITAMIN C WITH BIOFLAVONOIDS

1. *Angiology*, 1994; 45:566–73.
2. *Angiology*, 1994; 45:574–78.
3. *Diseases of the Colon and Rectum*, 2000; 43:66–69.
4. *British Journal of Surgery*, 2000; 87:868–72.
5. *Angiology*, 1997; 48:77–85.
6. *Journal of the National Cancer Institute*, 1999; 91:354–59

VITAMIN D

1. *New England Journal of Medicine*, 1998; 338:777–83.
2. *New England Journal of Medicine*, 1997; 337:670–76.

VITAMIN E

1. *New England Journal of Medicine*, 1994; 330:1029–35.
2. *Lancet*, 1996; 347:781–86.
3. *Lancet*, 1999; 354:447–55.
4. *New England Journal of Medicine*, 2000; 342:154–60.

VITAMIN K

1. *American Journal of Clinical Nutrition*, 1999; 69:74–79.
2. *American Journal of Clinical Nutrition*, 2000; 71:1201–08.

YOHIMBE

1. *Journal of Urology*, 1998; 159:433–46.
2. *Urology*, 1997; 49:441–44.
3. *Journal of AOAC International*, 1995; 78:1189–94.

ZINC

1. *Annals of Internal Medicine*, 1996; 125:81–88.
2. *Annals of Internal Medicine*, 2000; 133:245–52.
3. *Journal of Nutrition*, 2000; 1130:1512S–15S.
4. *Journal of Nutrition*, 2000; 130:1350S–54S.

SELECT BIBLIOGRAPHY

Blumenthal, Mark, et al., eds. *The Complete German Commission E Monographs: Therapeutic Guide to Herbal Medicines*. Boston: Integrative Medicine Communications, 1998.

DerMarderosian, Ara, ed. *A Guide to Natural Products*. St. Louis: Facts and Comparisons, 1999.

Duke, James A. *The Green Pharmacy: New Discoveries in Herbal Remedies for Common Diseases and Conditions from the World's Foremost Authority on Healing Herbs*. Emmaus, Pa.: Rodale Press, 1997.

Gruenwald, Joerg, et al., eds. *PDR for Herbal Medicines*. Montvale, N.J.: Medical Economics Company, 1998.

Jellin, Jeff M., ed. *Natural Medicines Comprehensive Database*, 2nd ed. Stockton, Calif.: Therapeutic Research Faculty, 1999.

Karch, Steven B. *The Consumer's Guide to Herbal Medicine*. Hauppauge, N.Y.: Advanced Research Press, 1999.

Lininger, Schuyler W., Jr., ed. *The Natural Pharmacy*, 2nd ed. Rocklin, Calif.: Prima Publishing, 1999.

Mahan, L. Kathleen, and Sylvia Escott-Stump, eds. *Krause's Food, Nutrition, and Diet Therapy*. Philadelphia: W. B. Saunders Company, 2000.

Peirce, Andrea. *The American Pharmaceutical Association Practical Guide to Natural Medicines*. New York: William Morrow and Company, 1999.

Tyler, Varro E. *The Honest Herbal: A Sensible Guide to the Use of Herbs and Related Remedies*, 3rd ed. Binghamton, N.Y.: Haworth Press, 1993.

Williams, Melvin H. *The Ergogenics Edge: Pushing the Limits of Sports Performance*. Champaign, Ill.: Human Kinetics, 1998.

ACKNOWLEDGMENTS

We wish to thank our editor at Henry Holt and Company, Deborah Brody, for her patience and good ideas; copy editor Muriel Jorgensen, for her careful eye; and our agent, Judith Riven, for playing matchmaker. Several other people helped out with the completion of this project more than they know. They include David August, M.D., William Hait, M.D., Joseph Aisner, M.D., Ann Gower, Cathy Gower, Alice Lesch Kelly, and Kelly Ormsby. Thanks for your insights and for listening.

INDEX

ABOUT THE AUTHORS

Dr. ROBERT S. DIPAOLA is a medical oncologist and associate professor of medicine at the Cancer Institute of New Jersey and the Robert Wood Johnson Medical School, located in New Brunswick, New Jersey. He cares for patients with cancer and conducts laboratory research and clinical trials. Dr. DiPaola is also the author of many research papers that have been published in leading scientific journals.

TIMOTHY GOWER is a journalist whose work has been published in many newspapers and magazines, among them the *New York Times*, *Health*, *Better Homes and Gardens*, *Reader's Digest*, and *Esquire*. His column, "The Healthy Man," appears monthly in the *Los Angeles Times*. The author of three previous books, Gower lives on Cape Cod with his wife, Ann.